TIME ALIVE

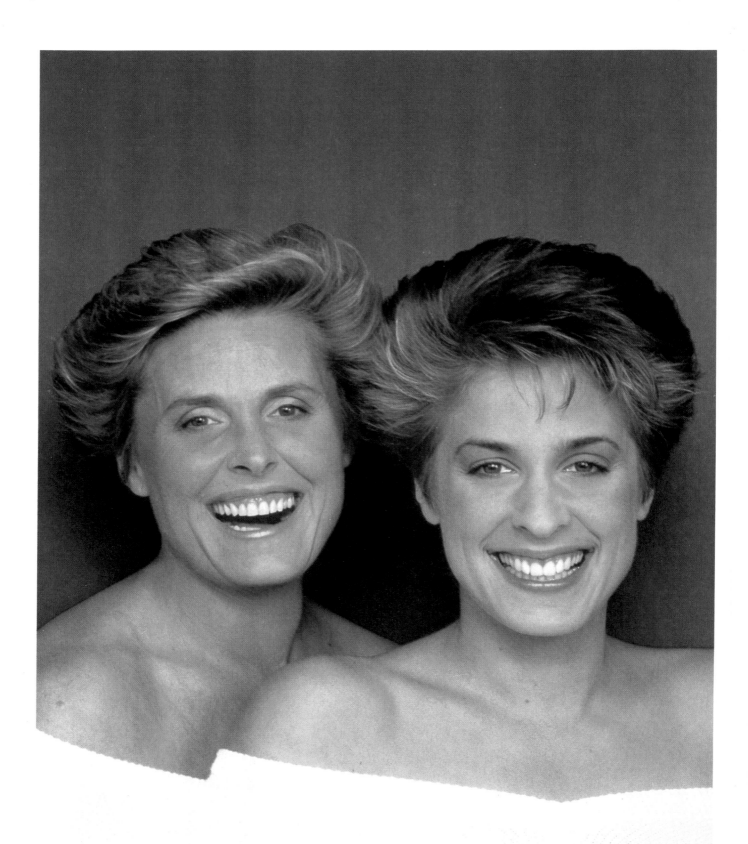

TIME ALIVE

Leslie and Susannah Kenton

Conran Octopus

Authors' Note

This is a book about wellness, not illness. The information in this book is intended for informational purposes only. None of the suggestions or information is meant in any way to be prescriptive. Any attempt to treat illness should come under the direction of a competent physician who is familiar with nutritional and exercise therapy.

First published in 1987 by
Conran Octopus Limited
28–32 Shelton Street
London WC2 9PH

Special photography of Leslie and Susannah Kenton by
Robyn Beeche and Carrie Branovan.

Art director   Tracy Drew
Designer   Karen Bowen
Design assistant Alan Marshall

ISBN 1 85029 083 0

Typeset by Tradespools Limited

Printed and bound in Hong Kong

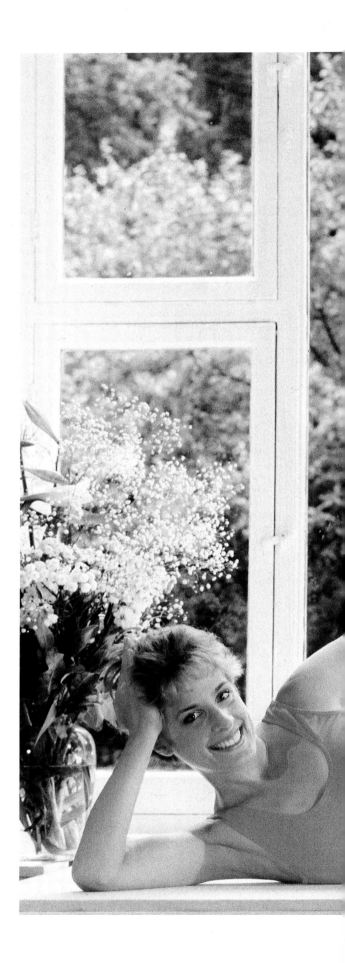

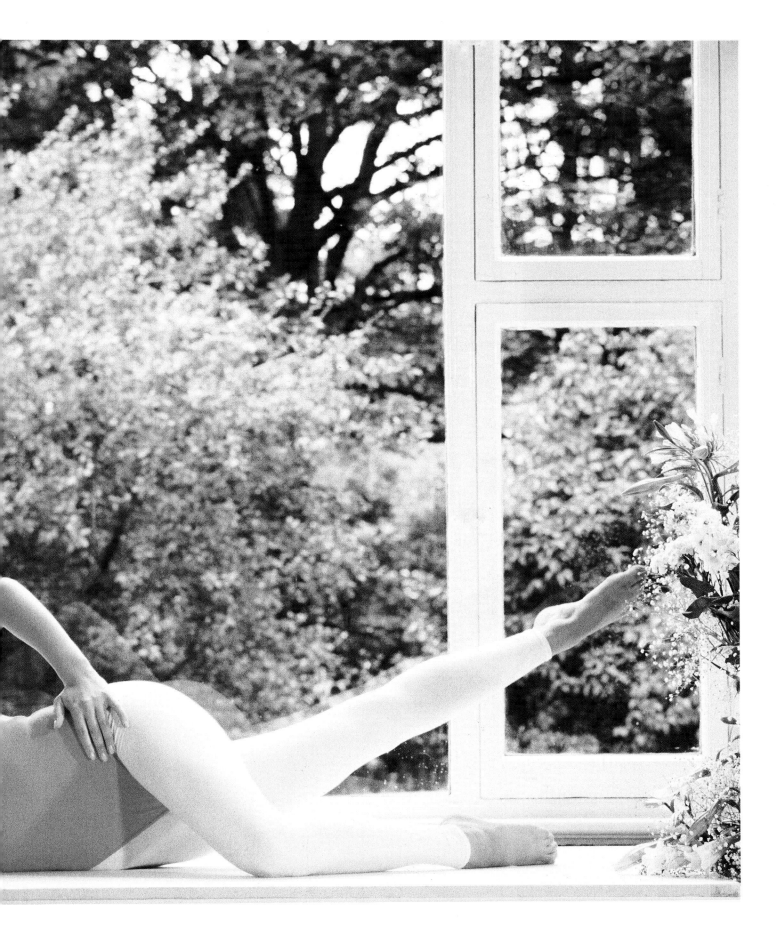

CONTENTS

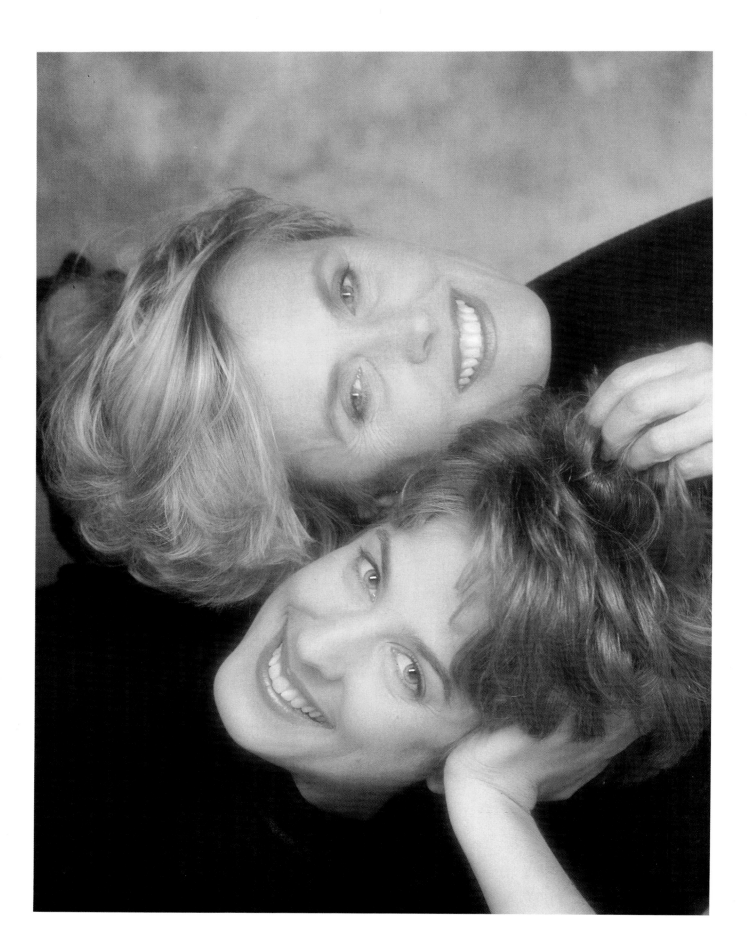

MAKING THE MOST
OF YOUR TIME ALIVE

The great mistake that most people make with a book like this is to treat it as something you should *slavishly* follow. Not at all. All of the tools for health and beauty, all of the techniques for helping you achieve high-level energy and mental clarity, all of the methods for self-knowledge – they are worth nothing in themselves. It is *you* who are important, *your* needs, *your* rhythms, *your* growth. The things you find in this book are *your* servants – not you, theirs. Make use of them, but have no fear of discarding any which don't work for you or have no meaning for you.

It is good always to remember that health in itself is not very interesting. It is merely the necessary foundation on which you can build your life – the creativity, the energy, the pleasure, the work. The things in this book are only bricks to help you build that foundation. Once it is built – once you have developed a life style for yourself that encompasses the needs of your mind and body and spirit, which allows all three to blossom – then you will worry very little about health again.

Your own barriers to energy and good looks will have been broken – beautifully broken. And you'll find yourself involved in a process of personal unfolding which is self-aware and self-regulating, so that when anything goes slightly wrong – you are fatigued or dispirited or confused – you will usually know from a kind of informed intuition what needs to be changed. To us, this is the most exciting thing of all about the *Time Alive* way of living – not having to think much about health and energy and good looks any more. You will simply *be* them.

By now, we have watched this unfolding process take hold in hundreds, probably thousands, of people who, like us, went searching for answers. We have seen it lead them to independence and autonomy and away from anxious worries about such things as what they should and shouldn't eat. Like us, sometimes they find it all a joy. At other times, they are faced with restrictions which need to be overcome. Like us, you will too. But the challenge of overcoming them brings its own excitement and its own rewards. And these challenges – whether they be physical, in relationships, at work, or spiritual – are always new and different. So long as you continue to wrestle with them, things get better and better. This is the crux of *Time Alive* – a process or a way of thinking and being which asks the very best of you and expects the same in return.

We both feel lucky to have shared so much of our own search for it with each other. In our learning and using all of the things which have gone into this book, and in the equally demanding task of finding ways of sharing it all with you, we have laughed together and fought with each other and struggled. We've felt the joy and the hopelessness, excitement and determination. We have also broken many of our own barriers for energy and good looks. And now we've learned to value the struggles as much as the successes. We know now that the hard times have been every bit as important as the moments of soaring spirits. So here we are. And now, like you, we each face our own *new* challenges. When we do look back, we know that the one thing we will never forget is the laughter.

Leslie

Susannah

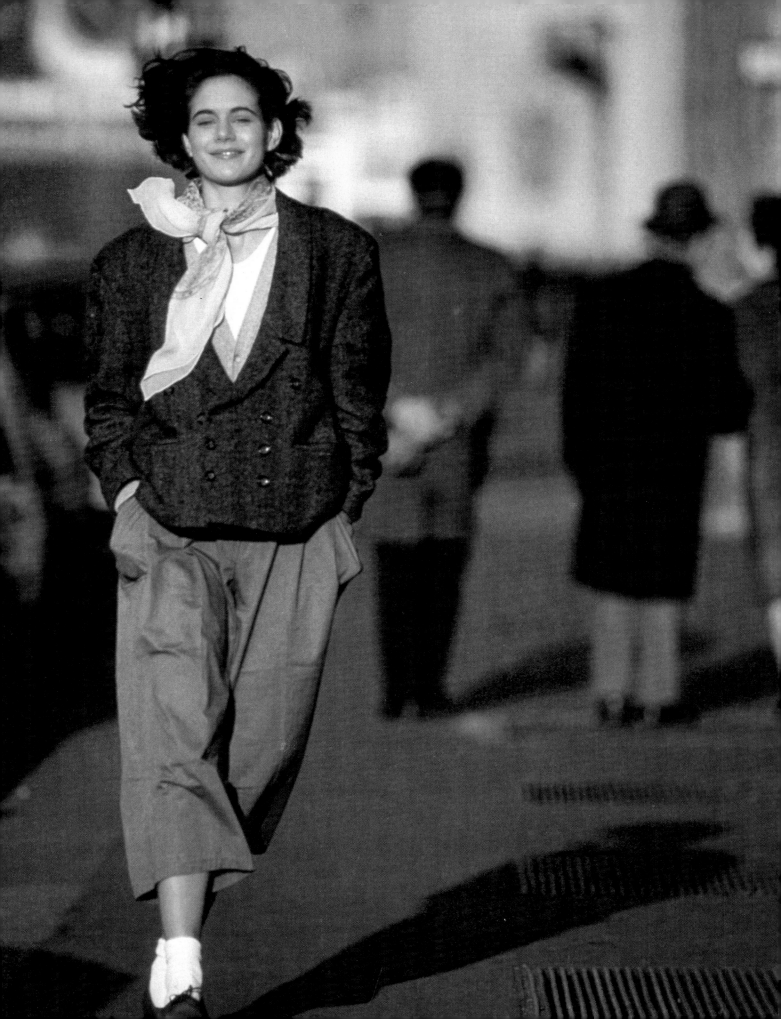

UP TIME

Lack of energy is the most common complaint of otherwise healthy people. 'I never seem to have enough energy,' they say, 'but what can be done about it?' Our answer might surprise you: we all have a great deal more potential energy than we ever use. The key to a high-energy life style is simply a question of learning to tap it.

Live each moment What, more than anything else, determines how much energy you have? It is not physical strength or what you ate for lunch or even how much you slept last night. It is simply whether or not you are totally involved at any particular moment in what you are doing – physically, mentally and emotionally. This is the finding of biologists, sports experts and psychologists who have studied the phenomenon of vitality and tried to distinguish between the traits of those people with high energy levels and the rest of us.

For a few lucky people the ability to live each moment fully comes naturally. For the rest of us it is something to be learned. We have to train ourselves in much the same way as students of aikido, Japanese sword fighting or tai chi – slowly and systematically. In Western society, we rarely function as a whole. Instead, we permit distractions to make the task in hand seem long and tedious and divide our concentration, with the result that energy is wasted. Learning to live each moment with total concentration on whatever you are doing is more than just a great way of creating energy. It is also the very best anti-stress trick you will ever learn.

On the physical side, there are also many tools you can use to revive yourself when you need pepping up, to banish fatigue and to call forth your energy reserves, such as certain energizing amino acids, specific essential oils with a stimulating effect on mind and body, aromatherapy and exercise methods.

Go for balance Maintaining a high energy level is all about balance. It is natural and good to be up some of the time and to wind down at other times. The trouble is that there are some times when it is more convenient to be up or down than others. Too often we treat ourselves like machines and ignore or over-ride the messages our bodies send to our brains. The result is a reduction of our sensitivity – our 'aliveness' – and consequently of our potential for work and play.

The *Time Alive* way is to tune into your body and listen to its needs. Once you understand the way it works and how it is affected by certain stressors, such as food or environment, then you can learn to choose your up times and down times. By maintaining a good balance between the two you'll never reach the stage of complete exhaustion that leads to serious illness.

RISE & SHINE

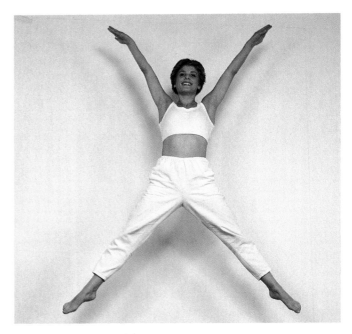

Getting out on the wrong side of the bed in the morning can leave you out of sorts for the rest of the day. Although the 'wrong-side-of-the-bed' syndrome has little to do with bed logistics or with chance, it does exist. How you feel when you wake up sets the tone for your entire day – for better or for worse. Whether you consider yourself a morning person or a morning grump, there is much you can do to improve the way you look and feel first thing, and hence throughout the day. Try the following routine to start your day on the right footing.

THE RIGHT-SIDE-OF-THE-BED WAKE-UP ROUTINE

● **Sweet dreams** One obvious key to waking up at your best is a good night's sleep. It is important to completely unwind from the stress of the day before going to bed, and for this a relaxation exercise can be helpful (try our Lovely Lazy Stretches, pp. 33–5). Make sure your sleep is not interrupted. For those who find it difficult to feel truly rested after sharing a bed for the night with a partner, it can be a good idea to have a separate bed to crawl into. If you do sleep in the same bed with a partner, be sure you have enough room and adequate coverings so you don't have to fight for the bedclothes.

● **Think positive** Before you go to bed, make sure you have a positive attitude towards the day to come. Set yourself a goal or challenge which you can look forward to fulfilling. You could promise yourself 10 minutes' more exercise than usual, or to get all your errands out of the way at lunchtime so you can go away for the weekend. Don't worry about what you have to accomplish, but look forward to the next day with optimistic anticipation.

● **Gentle wake-up** The wake-up alarm can be one of the most traumatic parts of your day. Some people insist that they simply won't wake up without an alarm that sounds like a fog-horn. Others rely on the wake-me-up-again-in-10-minutes type of alarm, which may go off five or six times before they actually get up. One of the most pleasant alarms is a clock radio tuned to a classical music station. It will bring you out of sleep gently, and help you step out on the right side of the bed.

The ideal wake-up alarm is your own internal clock. Provided you are not overtired or drugged, it should be very reliable. To develop your internal clock, try setting your alarm to a certain time and telling yourself you will wake up 15 minutes before it goes off. You will be surprised to learn how accurate your internal clock can become with a little practice.

● **Early morning exercise** First thing in the morning is our favourite time to exercise. If you are feeling a little sluggish, exercise can help vitalize your system and compensate for getting less sleep than usual. Even when you have stayed up very late the night before, it is worth waking up early to fit 15–20 minutes of exercise into your morning routine. Running and swimming are both good forms of aerobic exercise for those who live near a park or a swimming pool. Walking is also good. Rebounding, which is convenient and fun, has many health bonuses, and is one of our favourites. This is done on a mini-trampoline (or rebounder). You can bounce up and down, jog or do other exercises while listening to your favourite music or watching television. And because you do it in the comfort of your own home, you don't have to worry about bad weather or special gear or planning your whole day around it. All you need is a rebounder unit, some comfortable clothes and a little time (see our guidelines on pp. 21–3).

● **Freshen-up bath/shower** A warm bath or shower after morning exercise will help keep your muscles from aching. Before getting into the bath or shower, do a quick all-over skin brush (see pp. 96–7). A few drops of rosemary essential oil added to the bath water helps to invigorate you. After your bath, stand up and spray yourself with cold water from the shower attachment, or pour a jug of cold water over yourself. Then wrap up warm in a towel. Your body will feel tingly and glowing. If you take a warm shower, finish off with a cold rinse.

● **The high-energy breakfast** Give yourself the best possible start to the day by eating a light but sustaining breakfast (see pp. 14–15).

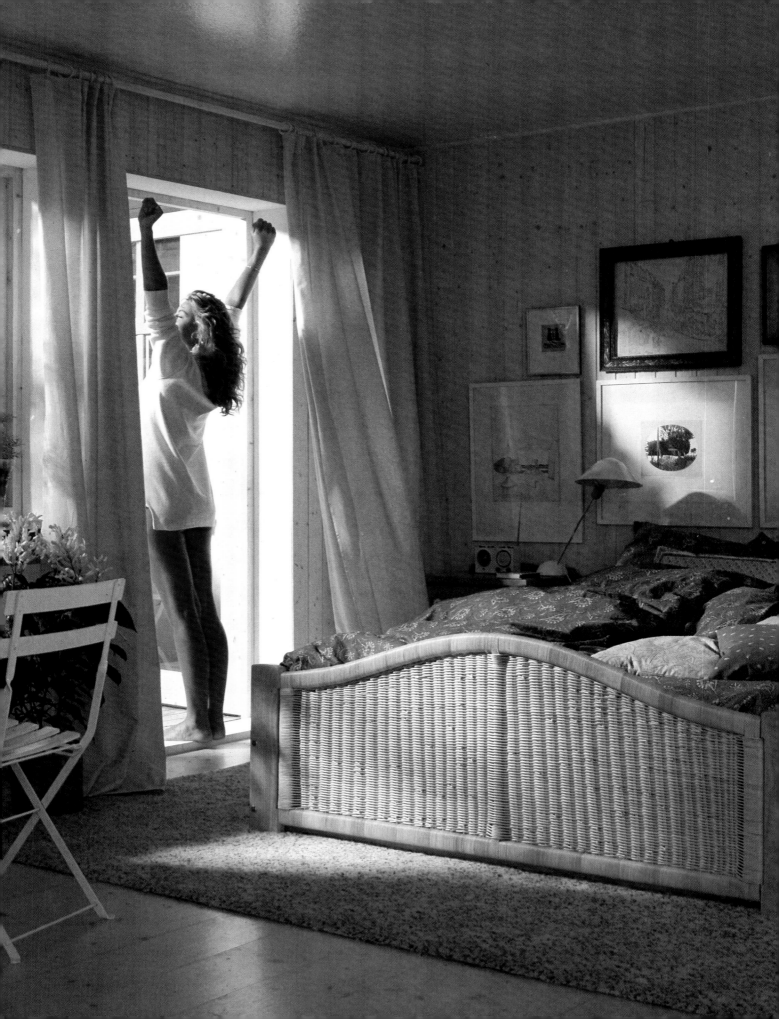

ULTIMATE BREAKFASTS

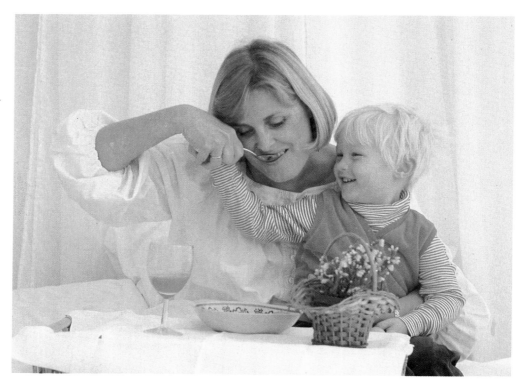

Two of our favourite high-energy breakfasts – Live Muesli and Energy Shakes – are made from foods which are easy to digest, are high in essential nutrients like vitamins, minerals and fatty acids, provide quick energy and will also help sustain you throughout the morning. If we have very little time, or if we ate a very large meal the night before, we often just have a piece of fruit for breakfast, such as an apple, a pear or a bunch of grapes. Fresh fruit is the ideal breakfast for anyone who wants to lose some weight.

WHY NOT A COOKED BREAKFAST?

A traditional cooked breakfast of, say, fried eggs, bacon, toast with butter and jam and tea or coffee is definitely bad news. In the first place, greasy food puts a great strain on your liver, which is working hardest to detoxify your body between midnight and midday, and its high fat content will leave you feeling tired and mentally dull. Secondly, such a breakfast is poorly combined, mixing complex proteins and complex carbohydrates, and contains mostly acid-forming foods, which means it will put unnecessary strain on your system and tend to make you feel jangly and stressed three hours after you've eaten it. Far better to choose an energizing breakfast, such as Live Muesli, an Energy Shake or fresh fruit.

● Live Muesli

This recipe is similar to the original muesli developed by the famous Swiss physician, Max Bircher-Benner. Unlike packaged muesli, which usually contains too much sugar, and is rather heavy and hard to digest, the bulk of this muesli is made up of fresh fruit. It will leave you feeling light and lively.

1–2 heaped Tbsp (15–30 ml) oat, rye or wheat flakes
a handful of raisins or sultanas
1 apple or firm pear, grated or diced
2 tsp (10 ml) fresh orange juice
1 small banana, finely chopped
2 Tbsp (30 ml) sheep's or goat's milk yoghurt (optional)
1 tsp (5 ml) honey or blackstrap molasses (optional)

1 Tbsp (15 ml) chopped nuts or sunflower seeds
½ tsp (2.5 ml) powdered cinnamon or ginger

Soak the grain flakes overnight in a little water or fruit juice to help break the starch down into sugars, along with the raisins or sultanas. In the morning, combine the soaked grain flakes and raisins with the apple/pear and banana, and add the orange juice to prevent the fruit from browning and to aid digestion. Top with the yoghurt, then drizzle with honey or molasses (if desired). Sprinkle with chopped nuts or sunflower seeds and spices.

You can prepare countless variations of Live Muesli by using different types of fresh fruit, such as strawberries, peaches, pitted cherries or pineapple, depending on what's available. When your choice of fresh fruit is limited, use soaked dried fruit, such as apricots, dates, more sultanas, figs or pears. For extra goodness, sprinkle the muesli with a tablespoon of wheatgerm. Wheatgerm, like unsulphured blackstrap molasses, is rich in minerals and vitamins (the B-complex vitamins in particular).

● Energy Shake
This recipe is delightful and quick – ideal if you have little time to spare in the mornings – and is best made from sheep's or goat's milk yoghurt.

8 fl oz (1 cup/225 ml) plain yoghurt
a handful of strawberries or raspberries
1 tsp (5 ml) honey or blackstrap molasses
1 Tbsp (15 ml) coconut (optional)
a squeeze of lemon juice

Combine all the ingredients thoroughly in a blender or food processor and drink. Depending on the type of yoghurt used, you may need to thin the shake with a little fruit juice.

As with Live Muesli, you can vary the Energy Shake by using different kinds of fruit, such as bananas, mango or fresh pineapple. You can also add extra 'goodies': a tablespoon of lecithin (especially good for slimmers), a raw egg yolk (good for hair and nails) or wheatgerm.

HOW TO FACE THE DAY WHEN YOU WISH IT WOULD GO AWAY

Feeling wretched after too little sleep, too much rich food and too much to drink the night before? The answer is to detoxify your system as quickly as possible.

DOs

○ **C/amino acid tonic**
For an unbeatable detoxifier, add 1 tsp (5 ml) powdered vitamin C and 1 tsp (5 ml) raw honey to a glass of gaseous mineral water. Drink this down with amino acid tablets: L-glutamine (500 mg), L-tyrosine (1000 mg) and glycine (500 mg). Repeat this tonic in 2 or 3 hours if necessary.

○ **Shiatsu**
When you suffer from a headache, drop your head forwards and place the tips of your fingers on the sides of your neck just below your ears. Using firm pressure, guide them back until they are 1 inch (2.5 cm) apart on either side of your spine at the back of your neck. Gently rotate your fingers there with firm pressure for about 1 minute. Repeat this 3 times.

○ **Breathe out**
Sit with your back straight. Breathe out, letting all the air escape. Breathe out even more again. Now let your abdomen swell, taking a deep breath in. Exhale immediately through your nose, pulling your abdomen in quickly so it forces all the air out. Relax your abdomen for a moment, then jerk it in again, releasing even more air. Repeat 6 times or until your lungs feel completely empty. Now take a long, slow breath in, hold it for a count of 5 and slowly exhale it all away. Repeat this whole exercise 6 times.

○ **Exercise**
If you have the time, take a brisk walk, go for a jog or do an aerobic work-out. Exercise is one of the best ways to eliminate unwanted waste from the body – through the lungs as you breathe and through the skin as you sweat.

○ **Water magic**
Hop into the shower and turn on the warm water until you are warm and tingling all over. Now change to cold water for 10–20 seconds, then back to warm. Alternate warm and cold – 2 minutes of warm with 30 seconds (never more) of cold – 3 times.

○ **Fruit breakfast**
A piece of fresh fruit with its natural sugar is ideal because it requires so little digestion. It will help detoxify your system still more. Take a good multiple B-complex vitamin as well.

DON'Ts

○ **Aspirin**
Analgesics cause a fall in blood-sugar and can upset your already delicate stomach – even in low doses.

○ **Coffee**
In your present state, drinking coffee is like flogging a dead horse. Each cup carries 80–120 mg of caffeine, which stimulates the central nervous system, pancreas and heart. Don't touch it now.

○ **Tea**
In addition to the unwanted stimulant caffeine, tea contains tannic acid, which can damage the mucous membranes of the mouth and digestive tract.

○ **Orange juice**
A drink of orange juice places additional pressure on the liver, already working hard at detoxifying.

EATING FOR ENERGY

There are no short cuts to eating well. The notion that you can eat whatever you like as long as you pop a few vitamin pills is simply untrue. We, too, have tried it and it doesn't work. Your way of eating largely determines whether you are brimming with energy or whether you drag through the day and evening, relying on coffee and sugar to get by.

The first 'do' for high-energy eating is actually a 'don't': never eat too much. Putting too much of even the very best food into your system will deprive you of vitality, because so much of your energy goes into digesting and assimilating the excess food and eliminating the wastes which are by-products of metabolizing it. Never eat when you are not hungry and always stop before you feel full.

GO NATURAL, GO RAW
The second key to eating for energy is lots of raw fruits and vegetables. For maximum vitality and good looks, 50–75 per cent of what you eat should be raw (see p. 27). A diet high in raw foods has been credited with stimulating healing, rejuvenation, an improved mental and emotional state and enhanced athletic performance.

Try cutting out all highly processed, ready-in-a-minute foods full of chemical additives. Then eat well on natural foods, such as fresh fruits and vegetables, wholemeal products and pulses or legumes, with smaller quantities of fish, game or non-factory-farmed poultry. Your energy levels will begin to soar.

SUGAR AND VITALITY DON'T MIX
Many people think that sugar provides energy, and much advertising feeds this illusion. True, sugar is high in calories, but these are largely empty. The energy jolt you feel after eating a chocolate bar comes from the sugar flooding into your bloodstream, which triggers the secretion of a hormone called insulin. It is the job of insulin to keep things in balance, so it encourages the sugar, not to be burned as energy, but rather to be stored as fat, thus reducing the level of your blood-sugar. So quick as a flash your energy vanishes.

Unfortunately, frequent sugar-eaters' bodies tend to over-react and lower the blood-sugar level too much. This is why the familiar (and very short-lived) lift in mood and energy which comes from eating a sugary sweet is soon followed by a depressive slump which can send you reaching for yet more sugar in a vicious cycle of fatigue and the effort to combat it. To avoid this high-low reaction and up-and-down cycle, steer clear of all refined carbohydrates – from sugar to white flour – and anything made from them. Instead, choose complex carbohydrates, such as fruit, vegetables and wholemeal breads and cereals, which release just the right kind of energy into your bloodstream slowly, bringing you sustained energy and enormous staying power.

Eating sugar also robs your body of chromium, an important mineral which stimulates the activity of enzymes involved in the metabolism of glucose for energy and the synthesis of fatty acids and cholesterol. Adequate chromium helps protect against chronic low blood-sugar and fatigue. Studies show that chromium deficiencies are common in Britain and the United States, in part because we eat so much refined sugar and in part as a result of agricultural practices which have depleted our soils of the mineral.

POTASSIUM POWER
If you are deficient in potassium, you are going to feel fatigued. More than any other single nutritional factor, a low level of potassium interferes with the high-energy life. Potassium is a catalyst in many cell enzyme reactions, including the essential biochemical process of glycolysis – the breakdown of glucose by enzymes to release energy. Potassium also looks after the activity of your nerves and muscles, and when too little of it is available you can become lethargic, weary and weak. It plays an important part in the conduction of nerve impulses, muscular contractions and cell membrane functions which ensure that your cells receive the oxygen and nutrients they need for high-level well-being and that their wastes are properly eliminated.

But potassium is easily lost from your body. Each day the average person loses about 7 per cent of his or her circulatory blood levels of the mineral through the urine. This means you need a fresh supply through your foods every day. Two factors contribute to potassium deficiency. First, potassium and sodium are antagonists which should balance each other in your body. Thanks to all the table salt added to convenience foods and used at the table to season foods, many people eat a high-sodium diet. Then sodium gets the upper hand, potassium levels drop and you can end up chronically fatigued. Low potassium levels also result from our Western tendency to eat too few fresh fruits and vegetables, which are high in potassium.

To increase your potassium levels, don't take supplements of the mineral, since most supplemental potassium – which comes in the form of potassium phosphate or sulphate – tends to pass unabsorbed through your body. Instead, increase your intake of fresh fruits and vegetables, their juices and homemade vegetable soups. Also, stop seasoning your food with table salt. There is plenty of natural sodium in wholesome foods without adding more. Three weeks of eating like this can dramatically heighten your energy level and increase your sense of well-being.

THE NUTRITIONAL UPPERS

Exploring the further reaches of eating for energy has led us to discover special 'energy-makers' – nutritional supplements which, when used together with healthy eating, leave you glowing and brimming with vitality.

● **Take C and see** Dietary supplements of ascorbic acid – vitamin C – have a remarkable ability to increase energy levels in many people. Just why this is so remains something of a mystery. We do know that the build-up of toxicity in the body depresses energy levels by causing free radical damage to cells and tissues (see pp. 108–9). Vitamin C is an anti-oxidant nutrient of the first order: it mops up free radicals, detoxifying the body and enabling you to tap your energy resources with greater ease. It is further claimed that high doses of vitamin C can help prevent arthritis, cure the common cold, slow down the growth of cancer cells and protect the body from air- and water-borne pollution.

But there may be more to it than that. Some experts contend that it is not a vitamin at all, but rather a unique substance which encourages energy transfer in the cells and tissues. If this is true, then ascorbic acid's way of increasing overall vitality parallels that of a high-raw diet: increasing cell vitality and use of oxygen, heightening the exchange of nutrients and wastes and generally stimulating cell metabolism. Like so many who value a high-energy way of living, we take a high-dose supplement, drinking about ½ teaspoon (1–2 grams) of pure vitamin C powder mixed with water or fruit juice with breakfast, lunch and dinner.

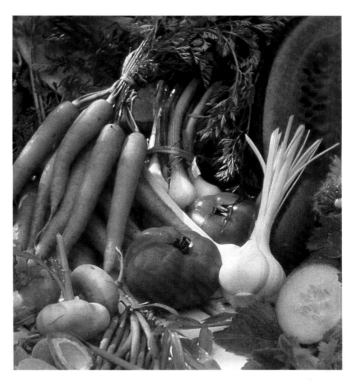

But is it safe to take this much vitamin C each day? Despite negative publicity in the past 10 years, there is no evidence that such doses are harmful. Some scientists worry that one might develop a dependency on this vitamin if it is taken in such high amounts. Soviet researchers recommend that you take high-dose supplements when you are stressed or for three or four weeks, then stop them for the same period of time. This is what we do.

● **The bouncy B-complex** If you are at all deficient in some of the B-complex vitamins, you can find yourself chronically fatigued. They play many important roles in the body, from helping your enzymes convert proteins, carbohydrates and fats into fuel for energy to stabilizing your nervous system and helping you weather the storms of stress. B vitamins are now used in the successful treatment of depression, insomnia, chronic fatigue and even certain forms of serious mental illness. It is important that you get plenty of the important B-complex by avoiding sugar, other concentrated forms of carbohydrates and too much alcohol – all of which rob your system of the B-complex vitamins – and by including in your diet plenty of wholemeal cereals and breads. If you are a meat-eater, it is good to eat fresh liver (preferably lamb's) once a week. There are also some good B supplements on the market. Taking only some of the B vitamins without support of the complete group may eventually lead to deficiencies in those neglected, so look for a well-balanced multiple supplement with, say, 50 mg each of B1, B2, B5 and B6, 25 mg of B3 and at least 400 mcg of folic acid, as well as choline, inositol, B12 and biotin.

MOVE INTO TOP GEAR

One of the best ways to draw on those elusive untapped energy reserves is to get into a daily physical discipline, such as a long walk or a run, come rain or shine. Or follow an exercise routine on tape or video, come what may, at the same time every day.

FROM DISCIPLINE TO FREEDOM

We find that when we are working hardest and sleeping least is when we need an exercise routine the most. Recently both of us averaged no more than four hours' sleep per night for a two-week period. Instead of lying about in bed at dawn to catch yet another 45 minutes of sleep, we got up half an hour early every morning and used the time to bounce on a mini-trampoline or run. This discipline made it possible for us to keep going under the demands of a strenuous work and travel schedule without excessive fatigue and without falling prey to minor infections, such as flu or colds.

Long-distance runners, cross-country skiers, hill-walkers and long-distance swimmers tend to be energetic, vital and positive people. This is because they regularly follow a physical discipline which demands sustained strenuous effort. Physical demands of this sort can only be met by entering an aerobic condition, a state in which outflow of energy is balanced by an increase in oxygen intake through deeper and fuller breathing. In the aerobic state the feeling of painful effort and struggle can be replaced by a sensation of effortless floating on air. This experience is by no means confined to top athletes. Anyone, regardless of age or condition, who is prepared to invest a little time and regularly use his or her body at peak levels can experience it. The results of such a discipline are improved general health, an increased sense of psychological well-being and an apparently endless supply of energy.

What physical discipline you choose is less important than the commitment to practise it regularly – at least four times a week, and preferably five or six – without fail, no matter what other demands are made on you. But, far from being some kind of sacrifice, to opt for this kind of discipline is really one of the biggest favours you can do yourself. It is a way of bringing mind and body together to maintain balance and sustained vitality when things get difficult. If you know that you can call on yourself to get up and go through your regular exercise routine no matter what, you can begin to apply this self-belief and self-confidence to other areas of your life.

The effects of such a commitment are more than psychological. Regular physical effort helps detoxify your body, ridding it of waste products that build up from stress and fatigue. It also brings about dynamic changes in the biochemistry of your brain, so that your whole view on life can improve. Instead of feeling sorry for yourself when the wake-up alarm rings so soon, you awaken and face the day as an exciting challenge, no matter how little sleep you've had. You also learn to take wonderfully refreshing catnaps whenever you have even 2 or 3 minutes to spare, say while sitting on a bus or in a taxi. Once you learn the trick, such mini-rests are a great way to recharge yourself.

When you first begin an exercise programme, you need to take things slowly. By starting gently and gradually increasing the length and intensity of your work-out, you will achieve good results and be encouraged to continue. If you overdo it at the beginning, you may injure yourself or just put yourself off the whole idea. Very soon after beginning regular exercise you will find it becomes a joy – almost second nature – and something you simply will not want to be without. You will actually become addicted to it, and to the high energy levels and great feeling it brings. But getting into the exercise habit demands a little effort at first, particularly if you have a poor image of yourself as someone who exercises. Both of us have been through this a few times, when force of circumstances or self-neglect have caused a breakdown in our exercise habits and we have had to rebuild them again from scratch. So pluck up your determination and get yourself in motion! Choose a physical activity – whichever you prefer, provided it is rhythmical and demanding – and practise it daily, or at least four times a week. Soon you will not be able to stay away from exercise, and the activity which required discipline at first will become easy.

PICK YOUR PLEASURE

The variety of activities you have to choose from are many. But be careful to differentiate between those which are aerobic and those which, because of their stop-start nature, are not. To be energy-producing, exercise must be steady and sustained. Anaerobic exercise, such as weight-lifting or isometrics, does little

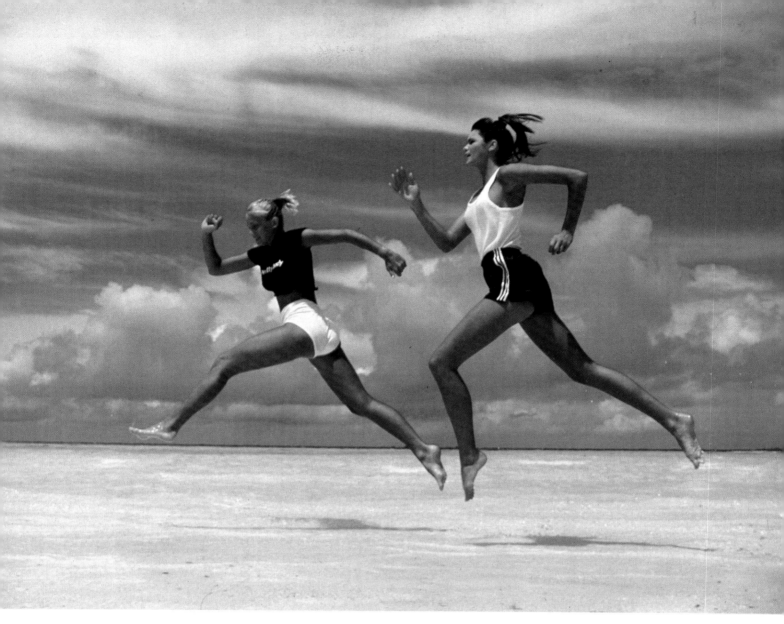

to stimulate vitality. Here is a list of various possibilities (by no means exhaustive) to give you some idea which are aerobic and which anaerobic.

● **Aerobic activities** Brisk walking, jogging, running, rebounding, cycling, dancing, skipping rope, skating, cross-country skiing, rowing.

● **Anaerobic activities** Squash, tennis, golf, downhill skiing, callisthenics, isometrics, weight-lifting.

● **It's got to be right for you** If you have the luxury of time to spare, then by all means do take up an aerobic form of dance or swim laps for 30–45 minutes each day at the nearest sports centre. But if, like most of us, you have many other demands on your time, then you will have to find other alternatives. One of the best ways to exercise is to begin your day with a long brisk walk in comfortable shoes. If you wear high heels at work, it is worth travelling to and from your office in a pair of flat walking or training shoes to exercise your leg muscles properly. Carry your dress shoes with you to put on once you arrive at work. If you have children and are housebound, get your partner to look after things for

half an hour while you go out for a walk or a slow, steady jog early each morning or when he returns in the evening. If your children are small, put them in a pram or a pushchair and take them with you – the extra effort of pushing them will do you nothing but good. Or consider buying a mini-trampoline and using it to bounce or run on the spot in your own living room while you look after your family, listen to music or watch television.

Whatever exercise you choose should fulfil the following criteria:

● It must be sustained and non-stop.
● It must last at least 30 minutes.
● It must keep your heart beating at about 70–80 per cent of its maximum capacity during the whole time you are exercising (see pp. 20–21). Exercising harder than this can lower energy levels, not raise them. If you want to get fitter faster, exercise longer rather than harder.
● It must be done at least four times a week.

TAP YOUR ENERGY

Every day, before you begin to exercise, raise your awareness of your body as an energy factory by focussing your attention at a point a couple of inches below your navel. This is known as the hara centre. The hara, located in the abdomen, has always been regarded as a well of power, like a smouldering furnace for ever ready to burst into the flame of activity. If you are able to imagine yourself emanating from the hara centre, you will experience a great release of vitality. This technique is traditionally used for creating powerful yet controlled movements for Oriental disciplines such as tai chi, aikido and even Chinese calligraphy. As you begin to exercise, continue to concentrate on this area and try to make every movement as though it comes from the hara centre.

Begin your activity slowly. Then, still focussing on the hara centre, gradually increase the speed and force of your movements. It is essential to find your own pace, which should be physically demanding enough to increase your breathing, but not be so demanding that you are left gasping for breath. You should feel that what you are doing is hard, but not a strain. If you feel any kind of chest pain, find yourself gasping for breath or become dizzy, then the effort is too great for your present physical condition, so slow down a little. Once you have found a pace that's right for you, you will be able to move in an aerobic state where you breathe fully and deeply without great effort or discomfort.

As you move, pay attention to your surroundings – the sights, the smells, the feel of the air – and to your own inner sensations. Visualize an object in graceful motion, such as a horse, an antelope or an eagle soaring in the sky, and imagine yourself as the thing in motion. It will give you feelings of strength and graceful ease which will help you to keep going. The whole experience should be demanding, exciting and satisfying. (But don't expect the excitement and satisfaction each and every time – nothing in life is that perfect.) When you feel you should stop, do. But be aware of why you have stopped. Are you short of breath? Anxious? Did you lose your image of motion?

MAKE IT A HABIT
Practise this energy-building trick for three weeks, letting your pace and images of motion change according to how you feel each day. Sometimes you will go faster, sometimes you will hold back. That is all part of life's rhythms. Simply be aware of what is happening and let it happen. But no matter what your mood or circumstance, continue your hara discipline. Gradually you will find that your body gains strength, your breathing comes easier and your movement becomes more graceful and fluent. At the end of the three-week period, your skin will look better (probably than it has for years), and you will find yourself bouncing with new vitality and radiating a healthy glow. Then your energy level, no matter what kind of energy you need at any moment – mental, physical, emotional – will begin to soar.

SAFE AND ENERGIZING
Whatever form of aerobic activity you choose, it should maintain your heart rate at about 70–80 per cent of its maximum. This figure, which is known as your 'training heart rate', is easy to determine.

● **Taking your pulse** To monitor your level of aerobic exercise, you will need to monitor your pulse rate. Find your pulse by laying your fingertips on the artery on the thumb side of your wrist. If you have difficulty finding your pulse in your wrist, try laying your fingertips against the side of your neck. When you have found it, count the number of heart beats for exactly 6 seconds and multiply this number by 10. The resulting figure is your pulse rate.

● **Finding your resting heart rate** Three or four times a day, take your pulse while you are sitting quietly for 6 seconds and multiply by 10. Add together all the pulse rates you have collected during the day and divide by the number of readings you have made to get your average resting heart rate.

● **Calculating your maximum heart rate** To determine your maximum heart rate, subtract your age from 220. Your maximum heart rate is the fastest your heart can beat at your age. (You must never exercise at this level!)

● **Setting your training heart rate** Your training heart rate is the ideal rate at which your heart should beat while you are carrying out your aerobic exercise activity. Calculate it by first subtracting your resting heart rate from your maximum heart rate. Then multiply the difference by 65 per cent ($\times$ .65) and add back your resting heart rate. This will give you your training level – the figure you need to remember and work towards.

For example, if you are 45 years old with a resting heart rate of 70, then calculations for your training level would go as follows:

Maximum heart rate: $220 - 45 = 175$

Training heart rate: $((175 - 70) \times .65) + 70 = 138.25$

In this case your training heart rate level should be around 138 beats a minute for maximum benefits from exercise. So when you are actually doing your aerobic activity – walking or rebounding or steady swimming or whatever – stop and check your pulse to see that it is just at this level. If it is 10 beats slower, then you need to make more effort. If it is 10 beats faster, slow down – you are working too hard and not getting your full fat-burning benefits from the activity.

As you continue to exercise over the weeks and months you will become more and more fit, with two results. First, your resting pulse itself will tend to drop as your heart becomes stronger and more efficient at delivering blood and oxygen to your cells and tissues. (Then you will have to recalculate and update your training level.) Second, you will continually have to work a little harder to keep your pulse rate at training level.

These are both wonderful signs that you are getting the very best out of your energetic life style. By the time you record your improved heart rate, you will already feel the difference yourself.

LOG YOUR PROGRESS

Keep track of your aerobic exercise by logging all the facts to make sure you are spending the time needed to make the most of its ability to stimulate fat loss and keep you at a very high level of fitness and energy. Set up a daily log book with a month devoted to each page. Record your present training heart rate at the top of the page and each day record the date, the form of exercise you have done, the time you have spent on it and your pulse rate as soon as you stop exercising. You can also make note of your weight and the measurements of your waist, your hips, your thigh and your upper arm at the end of each month. Even more important, at the end of each month write a few lines about your energy levels. Your log book will keep you aware of your exercise commitment and the results at the end of each 30-day period will delight and inspire you.

Rebound Rewards

Rebounding is an excellent form of aerobic exercise and one of the best to start with – good for strengthening your heart and lungs and firming your muscles. The unique up-and-down movement of your body on a mini-trampoline subjects it to changes in gravitational force. For a split second at the top of the bounce, gravity or G-force is non-existent – you are suspended in a state of total weightlessness like an astronaut in space. But at the bottom of each bounce, as you come down upon the elastic platform, the pull of gravity on your cells, muscles and tissues is suddenly increased by two or even three times the usual G-force on the earth. This puts your entire body – from the smallest cell to the largest bone – into a state of rhythmic pressure which can have beneficial effects on how you look and feel.

Such rhythmic pressure stimulates your lymphatic system – your body's waste disposal system. This encourages elimination of stored wastes from cells and tissues which would otherwise build up and lead to lowered vitality, the formation of cellulite and premature degeneration. And rebounding is so easy – the kind of exercise which anybody, from the severely overweight to the very athletic, can do, no matter what his or her current state of fitness.

Everyone can benefit from it. As your fitness improves, you simply have to work a little harder to get the same results in aerobic terms.

Many people, particularly those who wish to lose weight, start exercise programmes only to abandon them again within a few months. A high proportion of those who begin rebounding, however, regularly continue with it because it makes them feel and look so good, and because it is so much fun. You can quickly come to feel the exhilaration of the child who jumps for joy. And that, after all, is the highest experience you can get from any form of exercise – energy *par excellence*!

It is important to wear comfortable natural-fibre clothing, such as a cotton tracksuit, to allow your skin to breathe. Most women should also wear a good bra, and a well-fitted sports bra of the sort available from most sports shops and department stores is ideal. If you are new to rebounding or haven't exercised for a while, start by bouncing gently on the unit so that your heels only just leave the platform. If you feel unsteady, use the back of a chair to support yourself with your arms as you bounce. If you suffer from backache, go very gently and try to maintain a good posture as you bounce by directing the top of your head towards the ceiling. You should only bounce for a few minutes at a time. Try alternating small bounces with gently jogging from one foot to the other. As your strength improves you will be able to increase the height of your bouncing and also the length of time you exercise. Once you can bounce for 10–15 minutes without becoming breathless, incorporate exercises into your bouncing to help tone specific areas such as hips, waist, thighs, etc.

ADVANCED REBOUND ROUTINE

This whole routine should take 15–20 minutes. If you want to do a longer routine, simply continue to bounce after you finish the exercises for up to 45 minutes total.

Wake up and Warm up

When your muscles are cold it's not a good idea to do vigorous stretching out exercises in order to 'warm up'. Only do stretching exercises after warming up, otherwise you may injure yourself. Begin the rebound routine with 5 minutes of gentle bouncing to loosen up your muscles.

Jumping Jacks

Follow the warm-up bounces with 3–5 minutes of Jumping Jacks to really stretch your spine, lengthen your waist and tone up your arms and legs. Start with your feet together. Bounce them apart as you raise your arms up over your head so your hands come together. Then, as you bounce your feet together, bring your hands down to your sides.

Twister

Using your arms as a counterbalance, jump up while twisting your hips from side to side. As your leg twists one way, your arms and upper body will naturally swing the other. Do the exercise for 2 minutes. It will help trim your waistline.

Chest Toner

Continue bouncing and extend your arms out in front of you, making your hands into fists. Bounce and bend your elbows, pulling your arms back as if you were rowing. Bounce again, re-extending your arms in front. Each time you pull your arms back – on every other bounce – count 1. Repeat for 16 counts. This will help tone and firm your bust.

Arm Circles

In rhythm with your bouncing, circle your arms backwards for 16 counts then forwards for another 16. You have to move your arms quite quickly to keep in time with your bouncing. This exercise will help tone up the arms. Repeat the Chest Toner sequence again and then repeat the Arm Circles.

Can-Can

This and the following two kick exercises in combination will help you tone hips, abdomen and thighs. As you bounce, bend one leg up to your chest, bounce again on both legs and then kick the same leg out straight. The exercise should go bounce/knee bend/bounce/kick. Repeat 16 times, kicking alternating legs, with each straight leg kick counting as 1. Do the first set of kicks low and the second set a little higher. If you have a weak back, keep the kicks very low.

Side Kicks

These are similar to the Can-Can sequence, but you kick your legs straight out to the side one at a time. The exercise should go bounce/kick/bounce/kick on alternating legs. Repeat 16 times.

Cross Kicks

This exercise is especially good for the outer thighs and hips. As for Side Kicks, it goes bounce/kick/bounce/kick on alternating legs, but this time the leg bends at the knee and swings across the body. Lift the foot of the kicking leg so that its lower half comes parallel to the floor as you kick. Repeat for 16 counts. Bounce to catch your breath and then repeat a second set of leg kicks – Can-Can, Side Kicks and Cross Kicks.

High Bouncing

Finish with 5 minutes of vigorous bouncing or jogging, lifting your knees high.

top **Jumping Jacks**
bottom **Can-Can**
opposite **High Bouncing**

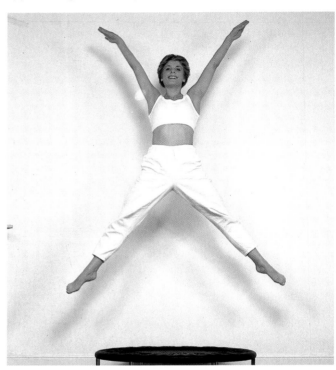

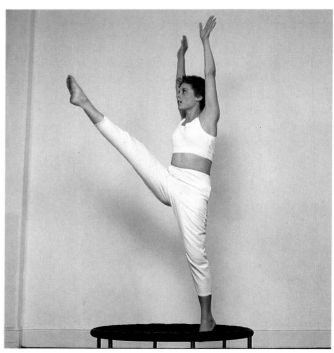

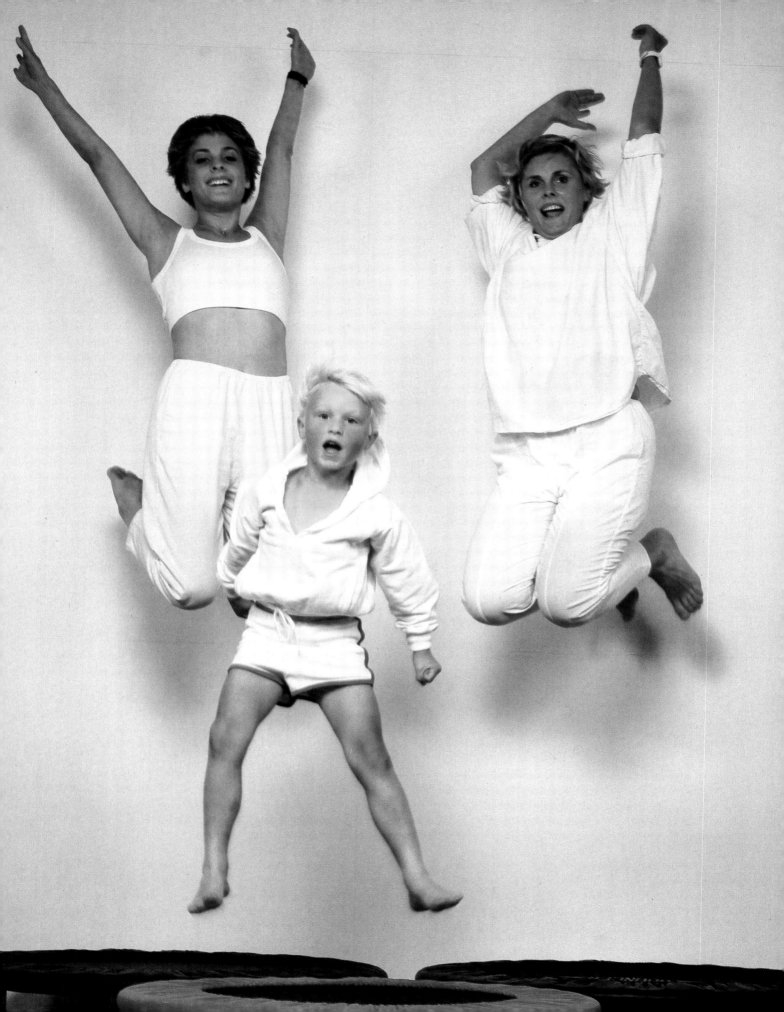

FOR THE LOVE OF ENERGY

Energy is a magic quality which depends on many interrelated aspects of your life – mental, physical, emotional. Get into energy and see how it feels. You will then invariably create more and more of it for yourself. Where there is energy, depression is absent, which is why regular exercise improves your mood.

RELEASING ENERGY

Loving creates energy. Negativity suppresses it. Even the simple habit of being direct and honest with people about what you think and feel leads to greater vitality. This is something we have both had to learn the hard way. It *is* possible to be both polite and truthful.

So what should you do when you are feeling low and in need of a boost? The first thing is simple – rest. Rest is a great energizer, and if you try to carry on for too long without it, you will deplete your long-term vitality. But in the short term, use quick energy tricks, such as aromatherapy or an energy breath technique (see opposite), to boost your reserves.

Each of us is born with different energy levels. Some have a gift of natural vitality, just as some people are born beautiful while others look average. But each one of us has far more energy in reserve then we ever use. Love is the key to releasing it. When you are doing something you love or are with someone you love, you tap energy resources better than at any other time. In fact, your energy levels are often superb indicators of how much you love life in general. After all, who wants to leave a great party at its peak? As much as you possibly can, do what you love. That is the first step in learning to love what you do. Both are high producers of lasting energy.

GET MOVING TO BANISH DEPRESSION

Several studies have shown that regular physical activity can help to overcome depression and fatigue. Richard Driscoll, an American psychologist, studied university students suffering from fatigue and stress-induced anxiety. Dividing them into groups, he gave one group standard forms of psychotherapy, another drug therapy and made a third group go running every day. At the end of the term he reassessed the groups and found that the daily runners' symptoms had improved the most – and they also achieved the highest exam results. Follow-up studies reach similar conclusions.

ESSENCES OF ENERGY

Essential oils of plants and flowers are perhaps the most beautiful of the quick energy tricks you can use to pep you up when you need it. These essences are not actually oils, but rather complex, highly volatile, natural hydrocarbons distilled from plants, which appear to retain some of the life force of the plants from which they have been gleaned. Chosen wisely and used when you need them most, essential oils act almost as catalysts for the body's own healing and restorative processes. The treatment is called aromatherapy. It can work magic to revive a tired aching body or a jaded spirit. Get to know the best essential oils for regenerating your energy and restoring you when you are tired and use them often (see pp. 36–7).

● **Footbath reliever** This is pure delight after a long day on aching feet. It helps relax and regenerate the whole body. Put five drops of pure essence of rosemary or bergamot into a basin of water slightly warmer than the temperature of the surface of your skin (so you can just feel the warmth). Sit comfortably with your feet immersed in the water for 10 minutes. Don't let the water get cold. If necessary, top it up with more warm water. Now dry your feet well and massage them with a good-quality almond, hazelnut or sesame oil. Put on a clean pair of socks and sit or lie for another few minutes with your legs elevated above your head. You will emerge from this simple treatment feeling like a new person.

● **Pep-up body massage** Make your own pep-up body massage treatment by combining the oils of basil, bergamot and geranium with a good carrier oil, such as sesame oil, in proportions of 15 drops of the combined essences to 3 tablespoons plus 1 teaspoon (50 ml) oil. Massage this oil all over your body (except your face) as soon as you emerge from a bath or shower. (There are nerve centres along the spine which respond well to aromatherapy, so if you can get someone to massage it up your spine for you, so much the better.) Rest for 5 or 10 minutes with your feet up.

● **Reviver bath** Add two drops each of bergamot, marjoram, sandalwood and neroli essences to a 100°F (38°C) bath. Climb in and stay there for 15 minutes, topping it up from the hot water tap when necessary to maintain the temperature. Then wrap yourself up in a Turkish bath robe or a big towel and lie down for 10

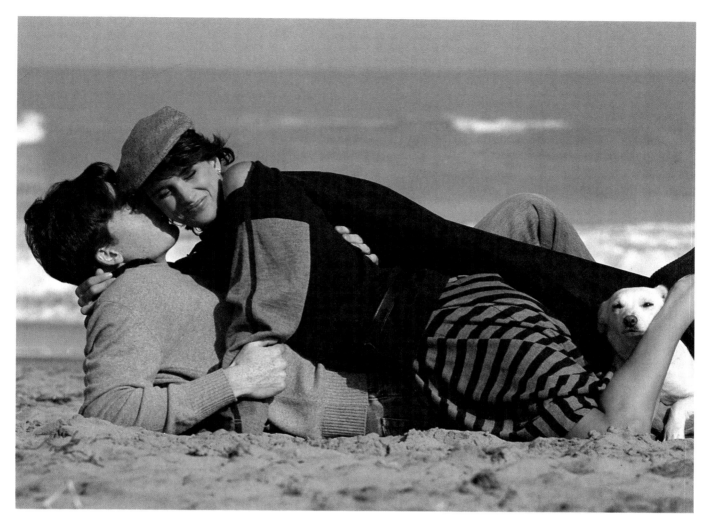

minutes. Another helpful trick in the bath when you are worn out is to get into a warm bath with essential oils and, once your body is warmed through, turn on the cold tap so that cold water just trickles into the tub and the temperature in your bath is slowly reduced to body temperature, which takes about 5 minutes. Then get out, wrap up well and lie down for 10 minutes. Either treatment works wonders for a tired body which needs access to its hidden energy reserves.

THE QUICK ENERGY BREATH

It is actually possible to breathe in energy. Try this for a couple of minutes: close your eyes and breathe slowly and deeply, imagining that you are breathing in vitality from the air to fill your whole body through the hara centre. As you breathe in, feel that your whole body is becoming more and more relaxed. Imagine it as a centre of immense light radiating outwards in all directions, as though you are taking in energy through the hara, transforming it into light and radiating it out again everywhere.

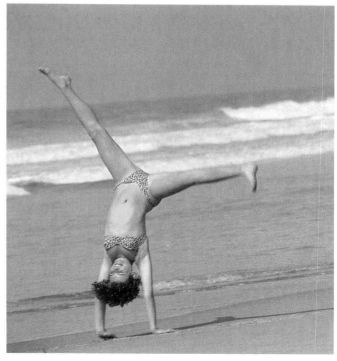

A HIGH-ENERGY LIFE STYLE

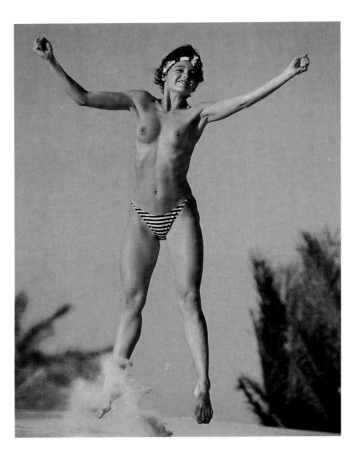

Living the *Time Alive* way doesn't mean rushing around in a manic state or being busy all the time. Far from it. Your energy, like the year, will have its seasons. There are times when it will be dynamic and others when it will be soft and tender. Some days you will use it to be brilliant or to battle against an obstacle which appears in your way. Other days your energy reserves will allow you to surrender yourself more wholeheartedly than ever before to the beauty of a piece of music or the abandonment of making love.

CONCENTRATED ENERGY

High energy the *Time Alive* way means, more than anything else, an ability to live fully, to give of your very best and to be open to all the good things life has to offer. In many ways it is a little like being a child again, where the colours are so vivid and the world is so full of wonder. Now is the time to take a look at your own energy habits and see if maybe some of them need changing. Then, gradually, you will be able to create for yourself a high-energy life style which in time will become second nature. Once you learn how to tap into the energy within yourself, once you experience how

good a high-energy life style can make you feel, energy will never again be something you have to worry about.

Worry and tension waste an enormous amount of energy. One of the most important steps in learning to use energy wisely is noticing when your energy is being frittered away unnecessarily. Are you putting it all into the task at hand? Or are you wasting it in anxiety, irritability or fear about failing in what you are doing?

Distractions and anxieties inhibit your full involvement in what you are doing and drain your energy unnecessarily. You can do something about them, either by changing your methods, place or type of work, or by refusing to pay attention to people or thoughts which are distracting you, concentrating all your energy instead on the task in hand. Next time you have something specific to do – be it mundane (such as your laundry) or unpleasant (such as your tax form) or demanding (such as increasing your physical exercise) – try taking the high-energy approach and see how you get on. Then apply it more and more to all the things you have to do until the distractions and anxieties have either disappeared or are being dealt with by a more positive and energetic you.

HIGH-RAW ENERGY

Fresh, raw fruits and vegetables contain the highest levels of vitamins and minerals in perfect balance, and are also rich in fibre. Even more important, they are living foods. Recent research into the living cell leads scientists to believe that fresh foods are not only biochemically superior to their cooked and processed counterparts, but that they also may promote vitality in those who eat them, thanks to their subtle electrical or electromagnetic properties.

We vary the proportion of raw foods in our diet almost entirely according to the amount of stress we are experiencing at any given time. If we are worried or working long hours or exercising a great deal, then we will eat even more than 75 per cent of our foods raw. When we are relaxed or on holiday, the proportion will drop to 60 per cent or less.

Begin by making one daily meal a beautiful raw salad based on myriad crunchy, colourful vegetables. Eat it together with chicken, chopped egg or sunflower seeds. In two weeks you will feel and look so much better that you will quite naturally and without any special effort want to increase further your proportion of raw foods.

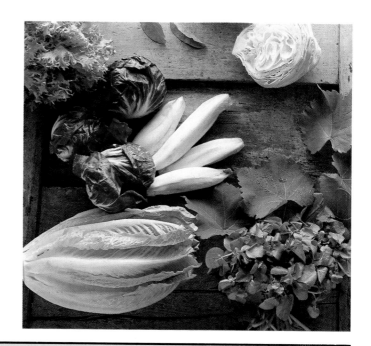

TEN KEYS TO THE HIGH-ENERGY LIFE STYLE

○ **Love life**
Energy begets energy. The more active your mind and body, the more energy you will call forth from your vast untapped reserves. Be creative in what you do and try to do what you want to do as much as possible. Nothing sustains energy better than the satisfaction of doing what you love and loving what you do.

○ **Get physical**
Regular aerobic exercise pumps up your vitality more than any other physical activity. It creates more oxygen-carrying haemoglobin in your red blood cells, increases the flow of blood through your veins and capillaries to nourish cells, and improves your muscles' ability to burn oxygen and calories.

○ **Toss out the sugar**
Eating sugar robs you of the nutrients necessary to keep your metabolism ticking over. It may boost your energy for a time, but it soon lets you down with a crash. Escape from the sugar trap and you will find your energy levels soaring.

○ **Use the water trick**
Alternating warm and cold water – in the shower, or splashing your face at a basin – is a great way to revive your flagging spirits and regenerate a tired body. Use it often.

○ **Shed your excess fat**
If you are carrying around more than 10 pounds (4.5 kg) of excess fat, you are undermining your energy potential. Get rid of it through regular exercise and altering your eating habits.

○ **Try the C trick**
Extra supplements of vitamin C can increase energy levels by detoxifying your system and improving the efficiency of your metabolic processes. Studies show that people deficient in ascorbic acid get tired more easily than those who have a high intake of it.

○ **More fruit & vegetables**
They are high in potassium – the anti-fatigue mineral which keeps you going long after others have dropped by the wayside. You need lots of potassium for the high-energy life style. Most of us eat too much sodium from table salt and processed foods, leading to depletion of potassium and, eventually, chronic fatigue. Season your food with fresh herbs instead of salt.

○ **Brighten up your looks**
When you feel down or fatigued, pick up your make-up brush and work some quick wonders on your face. Changing even a superficial thing like the colour of your blusher and making sure you are skilfully made up (which can be done in a matter of only a few minutes) will not only have you looking good, but will also brighten the way you feel and bring you access to greater energy.

○ **Take a break**
If you are already somebody with a tendency towards a high-energy way of life, make sure you give yourself time to restore all that vitality you give out day after day. Take a periodic break for a day or two to relax – read, listen to music or follow any other pleasurable pursuit you like. It will bring you renewed creativity and leave you sailing high with vitality.

○ **Be positive**
Nothing drains energy more than moaning – or having to listen to a moaner. Your consciousness is highly responsive to what is fed into it. If you project negativity to those around you, negativity will reflect back to affect you and you are likely to find yourself drained of vitality. Misery, like happiness, is contagious. Try to be a sunshine type and not a moper. Be careful, too, about how you choose your friends. For high energy, you should really like those with whom you spend your time, so avoid hangers-on or trendy people you believe you *should* like.

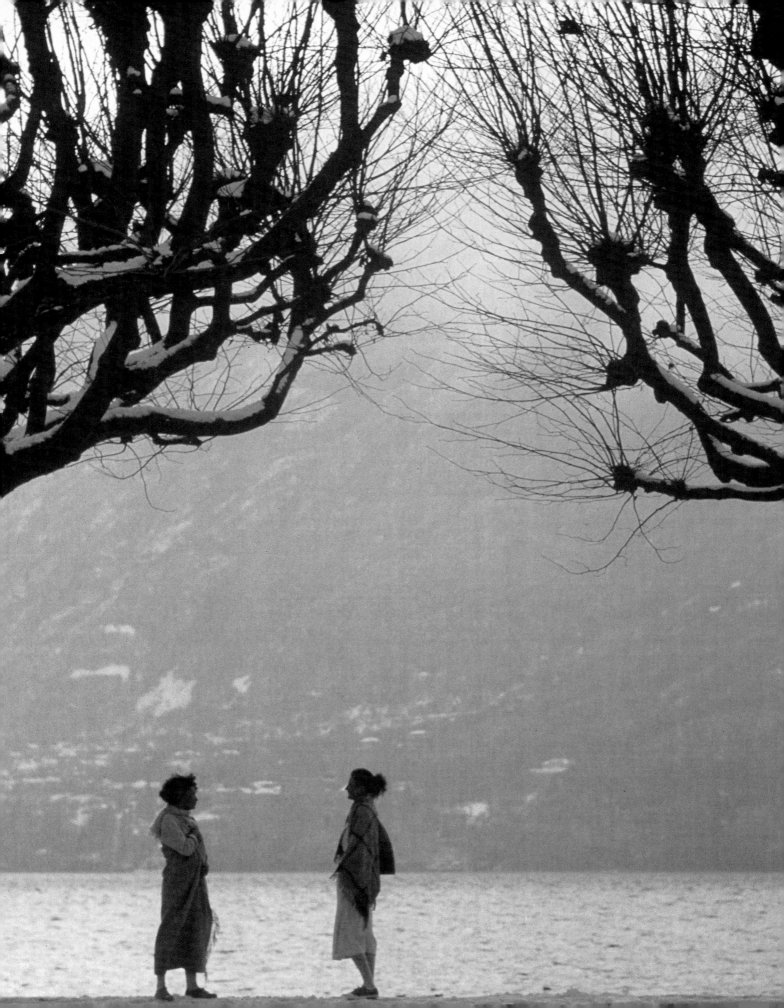

DOWN TIME

'What goes up must come down,' the saying goes. These few words should be engraved on everyone's brain – particularly those of us who opt for a high-energy life style. To experience high energy in a healthy way – not by taking drugs, drinking coffee or burning yourself out with stress – you must be able to let go, and to do so completely at will. That is something that most of us have to learn. After all, urban, 'civilized' society is not the best possible environment for keeping in touch with life's natural rhythms. Yet acknowledging these rhythms – from alterations in light and darkness to the need for balance between out-flowing energy and restorative in-flowing energy – is central to maintaining high-level vitality. It is part of making stress your friend, not your foe, and learning to cultivate deep relaxation as a tool for regenerating your energies, healing your body, calming and clearing your mind and bringing you a sense of joy and serenity to balance the excitement of being on the go.

Positive stress is not a bad thing. On the contrary, it is the spice of life, the exhilaration of challenge and excitement, the 'high' of living with heavy demands. But to make stress work for you, rather than against you, you must learn to let go of it when you need to. Stress and relaxation are two sides of the same coin. Learn to move easily from one to the other and you will begin to experience your life in terms of satisfying and enriching change, like the ebb and flow of the tides. Then you will avoid getting stuck in a highly stressed condition which saps your vitality, distorts your perceptions and leads to premature aging and chronic illness. 'Down time' is not merely a helpful adjunct to the high-energy life style – it is absolutely essential to it. It brings great bonuses too, since most of the tools and techniques for helping you to experience it are sheer delights to use.

GETTING THE BALANCE RIGHT

Stress is a fashionable word. We worry about it, wonder about it and wish it would go away, usually without even stopping to find out what it is. In fact, stress is a simple biological phenomenon with specific biochemical characteristics. It occurs whenever your body is really challenged and is forced to rise to the occasion. This physical challenge can arise from emotional causes, such as being stuck in traffic or shouted at by your boss or a loved one, as well as from physical causes, such as over-exertion or living in an environment where air, water and food are polluted by chemicals.

Whatever its cause, there is no reason to fear stress. Indeed, people who learn to make the very best use of stress tend to *enjoy* its excitement. The trick to living well with stress and preventing it from becoming destructive is simple: make sure the stressed state is well balanced by consciously practised deep relaxation from meditation, exercise, good sleep and recreation. Then stress will be a good friend and you will learn to like it when it comes. As always, balance is the key.

When you are in stress, the action of the sympathetic branch of the autonomic nervous system comes into play; when you are in a state of relaxation, the parasympathetic branch is dominant. In almost every respect, the balance between the physical experience of relaxation and stress is perfect:

PHYSICAL INDICATORS	STRESS	RELAXED STATE
heartbeat rate	raised	lowered
blood flow to muscles	increased	decreased
blood flow to organs	decreased	increased
demand for oxygen	increased	decreased
cortisone output	increased	decreased
blood pressure	increased	decreased
muscle tension	increased	decreased

The result of these physical realities is that, in stress, your body is ready for action; in a relaxed state, your organs and systems function properly.

DIET MATTERS
Balance is important in terms of diet as well. When you are under stress, your body tends to produce many acid waste products, just as it does if you live on a diet high in sugar and meat. Eating a diet high in raw fruits and vegetables tends to alkalinize your system with alkaline substances, which helps keep you calm even in chaos. To sustain your vitality and keep your cool even at the worst of times – after a sleepless night or when you have been working very hard – make sure to increase the amount of raw foods in your diet and spend at least a few minutes doing a deep-relaxation exercise (see pp. 136–7). They can often keep you going even at the worst of times.

ANTI-STRESS HELPERS
Constant stress tends to deplete your body of specific substances which, when supplied in extra amounts for a short period, help you regain your balance and resist stress-caused illness. There are a number of good anti-stress vitamin tablets on the market, and a typical one would contain the following mixture of vitamins, minerals and other substances. You would want to take such a formula two or three times a day.

SUPPLEMENTS	AMOUNTS
B1	75 mg
B2	75 mg
B3	50 mg
B6	50 mg
Pantothenic acid	50 mg
Folic acid	400 mcg
Bl2	25 mg
Bl5	30 mg
Choline	50 mg
Inositol	250 mg
PABA	50 mg
Biotin	50 mcg
Calcium	1000 mg
Magnesium	500 mg
Zinc	25 mg

Vitamin C is also needed in extra amounts when you are under stress. We take the above formula twice a day, along with an extra 3 to 6 grams of vitamin C.

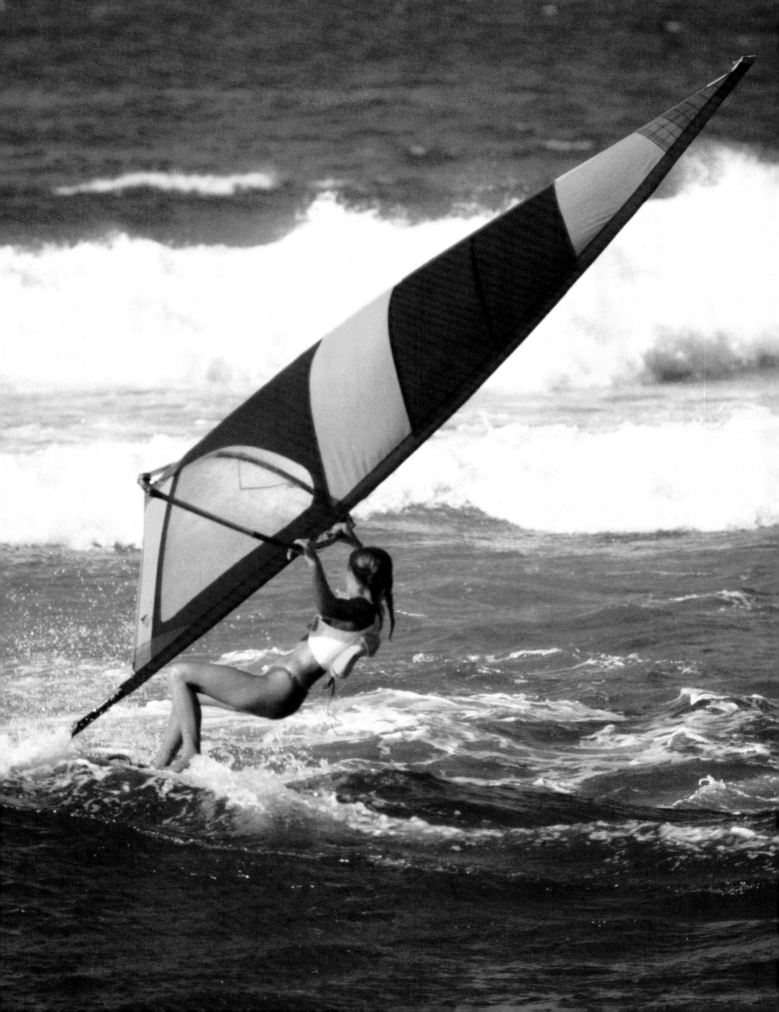

WINDING DOWN FROM WORK

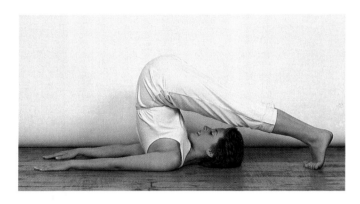

Arriving home from a long day's work can be the lowest point in your day. You stagger through the front door, sigh with relief and suddenly realize how overwrought you feel. A constant flow of adrenalin and the things you have had to do have kept you going all day, but now you're ready to collapse with nervous exhaustion. Perhaps you go straight to the refrigerator and begin sampling snack after snack – hoping eventually to find the magic food which will calm and restore you. Or you may collapse in front of the television and sit through a programme you hate because you haven't got the energy to change the channel.

DE-STRESS BY DESIGN
Winding down after work is just as important as energizing yourself for the day in the morning. Start by recognizing the signs of stress, such as muscle tension or a voracious appetite. Then make a conscious effort to de-stress. If you are hungry when you come in, don't just eat whatever you can find: a poor combination of food groups will put even more stress on your body and exhaust you even further. Rather, eat a piece of fruit to tide you over until dinner. Also, eating when you are nervous will not help your digestion and may leave you feeling bloated and headachy. Treat yourself to one of the following 'down time' de-stressors each day after work or whenever you need to calm yourself and let go.

STRETCH OUT AFTER WORK
Some people find that half an hour's aerobic exercise straight after work is just what they need to shake off work-time worries and supply a new burst of energy. If aerobic exercise seems too energetic, try our Lovely Lazy Stretches routine (see pp. 33–5) – a few simple stretches which rely mainly on the forces of gravity – so that all you do is let go and breathe. There's no jumping around or forcing your fatigued body to do umpteen sit-ups. You'll be surprised how much doing these simple exercises for a few minutes a day can improve both the way you look and feel.

WHAT CAN STRETCHING DO FOR YOU?
● **Relieve stress** Stress and anxiety become built into our bodies as permanent muscle tension. When you are in a difficult situation, your body readies itself for the 'fight or flight' response, and its muscles contract in preparation. Then, once the situation is over, you forget to let go and the muscles remain tense. Gradually this response to stress becomes a norm, so that you don't even know you are tense. The result is restriction of movement and loss of youthful agility.
● **Give you more energy** Your muscles consume a lot of energy maintaining a state of permanent contraction. If you can release the contraction and allow the muscles to relax, then you can use the spare energy for better things.
● **Improve your body tone** Muscles work in antagonistic pairs: when one is contracted, the other is relaxed. When a muscle is permanently tensed its antagonist becomes flaccid and bulgy, and undesirable physical distortions develop, such as a bulging stomach and thighs, a sagging bottom or a 'dowager's hump' at the base of the neck. Once you release tightly contracted muscles, the flaccid ones have a chance to tone up and your overall body tone will benefit.
● **Improve digestion and metabolism** Muscles are responsible for holding our internal organs in place. Well-toned muscles provide better support and thus assist the functioning of all our vital organs.
● **Cleanse your system from inside** When a muscle is stretched, the blood is squeezed out of it through tiny capillaries. When it relaxes again, fresh blood flows into it. This action removes wastes and brings nutrients and oxygen to the muscle.
● **Restore youthful grace** Ridding yourself of extraneous muscle tension and toning up flaccid muscles helps to improve the alignment of your whole skeletal system. This improvement of your posture means that you naturally move with much more grace and ease.

Down Time

THE LOVELY LAZY STRETCHES

These stretching exercises should not be done right after a meal, as they may interfere with digestion. Choose a time when you can be alone to enjoy them and relax. If you like, stretch to the sound of gentle music.

Repeat this series of stretches every day, or choose one or two to do whenever you feel tense in a certain area.

WALL PRESSES

These exercises use the force of gravity and a wall to stretch out the muscles of your neck, shoulders, back, legs and ankles.

Shoulder Press

Stand 3–4 ft (.9–1.2 m) from a wall, arms at shoulder width, and place your hands against the wall 2 ft (.6 m) above your head. Lean on your hands, letting your head and neck drop forwards and your chest sink downwards so that your back is bowed. Rotate the upper arms gently so that you don't hunch your shoulders. The stretch should last about 30 seconds. *Bonuses*: Helps relieve tension in common problem areas – the neck and shoulders.

Upper Back Press

Stand in the same position, and lift up your head and buttocks so that your back arches. Press the elbows towards the wall. Again, work the stretch for 30 seconds. *Bonuses*: Relieves pain and tension in the upper back and between the shoulder-blades, and helps break the hunching habit.

Heel, Calf and Hip Press

Stand about 1 ft (.3 m) away from the wall and put your arms straight out in front of you, level with your shoulders, and your hands against the wall. Place one foot back about 2 ft (.6 m) and press the heel towards the ground. You should feel the muscles in the back of your calf and heel stretch. By tilting your pelvis forwards you can also stretch the front of your hip. After 30 seconds, change to the other leg. *Bonuses*: Stretches out the calves and hips which get tight from a lot of walking and from wearing high heels all day.

Wall Splits

Sit on the floor parallel to the wall, legs extended in front of you, with one hip against the wall. Now lie down, swinging both legs up in an arc along the wall as you turn your body around so that you end up in a 'V' shape. Let your legs fall gently open with the force of gravity as far as is comfortable. (As you relax into the stretch and exhale they will open wider.) Extend your arms out to the sides parallel to the wall and allow your whole back to widen and lengthen against the floor. Stay in the stretch for 2–3 minutes and then gently roll out of it. *Bonuses*: Helps tone heavy thighs and relieves tension in the pelvis that can dull your sexual responses.

FLOOR WORK
Twist-overs

Lie on your back on the floor with your knees bent. Take a few easy breaths and feel your back lengthening. Cross your legs, left over right, and tuck your left foot under your right calf. Extend your arms out to the sides. Now slowly drop your knees over to touch the floor on the right side. Turn your head to the left. Stretch out your left arm and try to get your shoulder to reach the floor. Continue for 30–60 seconds and then return knees to centre. Hug them into your chest with your arms to relax your lower back. Repeat the exercise on the other side and then repeat both sides again. *Bonuses*: This exercise is for the waist and spine. Eases ache of the lower back by relieving pressure on the spine. Also helps trim the waist and increase shoulder mobility.

Lie Back Thigh Stretch

Kneel on the floor, sitting back on your heels. Unless you are very supple, place a cushion or two behind you to lie on; with practice you may be able to remove the cushions and lie back on the floor. Move your legs apart to create a space to sit in, but don't worry if you can't sit right down between your legs. Place your hands behind you and gradually walk them backwards. Gradually ease yourself further down, supporting yourself on your hands or forearms and making sure that your pelvis is tilted forwards so that you don't strain your lower back. *Bonuses*: This position helps relieve any menstrual problems, as well as tone the thighs.

Neck Rocking

This is a good preparation for the yoga Plough position, which otherwise can be a little uncomfortable if you go into it without this warm-up. Kneel down and rest the top of your head on the floor in front of you. Gently rock forwards and backwards over your scalp, feeling the stretch in your neck and upper back. Continue the exercise for 1 minute. *Bonuses*: Releases tension in the neck and massages the scalp to help promote healthy hair growth.

The Plough

Lie on your back. You may want to place a rolled-up hand towel or sweater under your neck for comfort. Bring your knees up to your chest and extend your legs up towards the ceiling. Allow your legs to drop over your head and let the weight of gravity bring them gradually down. The aim is to drop your feet all the way to the floor behind your head. Continue the stretch for 1 minute and then slowly roll your legs back down again, feeling each vertebra roll against the floor. Rest for a moment, lengthening out your spine along the floor, then repeat the stretch. *Bonuses*: Good for the digestive system and the thyroid gland. Also relieves tension throughout the back and neck.

Roll-up

Assume a crouching position with your feet comfortably apart, dropping your heels as close to the ground as possible. Hang in this position for 30 seconds, then place your hands on the floor in front of you and lift your bottom up towards the ceiling, straightening your legs if possible, but not straining. When your legs are straight, gradually roll up through the spine until you are standing. Stand tall and take a few deep breaths, feeling the relaxation in your muscles and ease of your posture. *Bonuses*: The crouching position is particularly helpful for constipation, and the Roll-up gives the whole body a general feeling of renewal.

For illustrations of the Lovely Lazy Stretches, see overleaf.

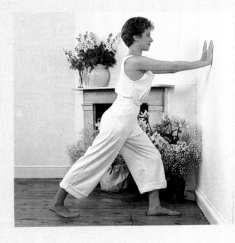

HEEL, CALF AND HIP PRESS

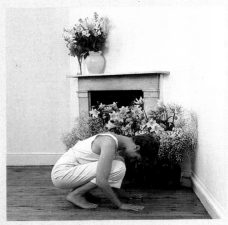
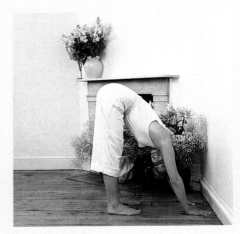
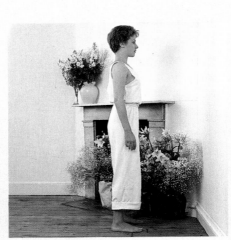

ROLL-UP

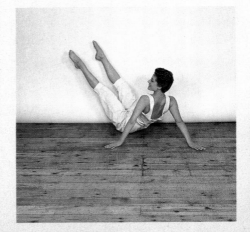
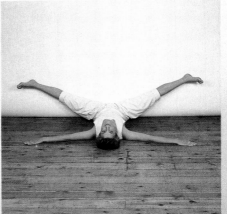

WALL SPLITS

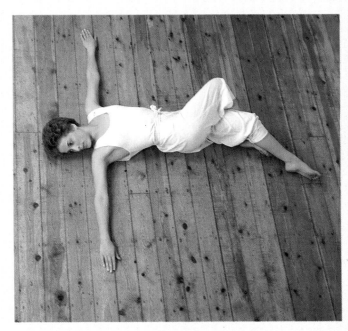

TWIST-OVER

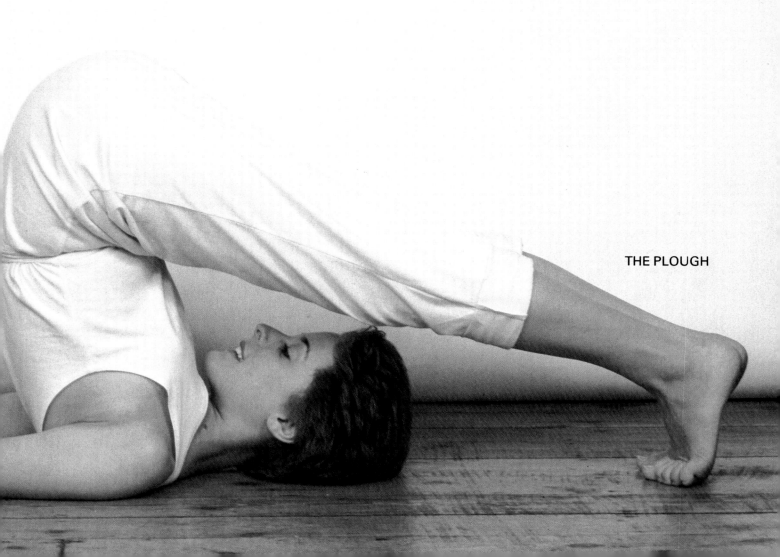

THE PLOUGH

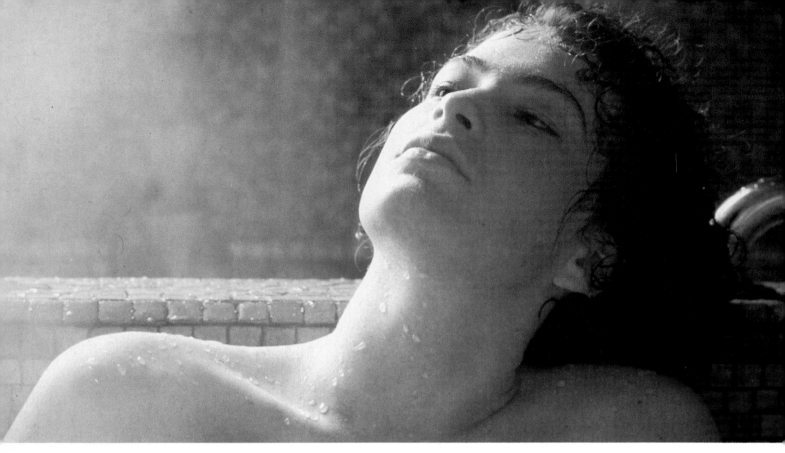

THE BENEVOLENT BATH

In a world where the benefits of an invigorating, quick shower are more and more appreciated, it is easy to forget the bliss of a long lazy bath. Water – especially when it has been fortified with plant essences – has the power to soothe, heal and relax a tense body and to lift a fatigued spirit. We don't take relaxing baths often, but we find them a godsend when we feel strung out or whenever we have particularly neglected ourselves. Then we take the telephone off the hook, put a Dvořák string quartet on the cassette player and head for the bathroom. We also find it an excellent way to ease aching muscles after running.

MIND-POTIONS
Allow an hour for the whole process from beginning to end. Make sure you have everything you need – towel, loofa or hemp glove, another towel to use as a head-rest and whatever plant essence you want to use. Each essence has a different effect on the mind and body. We have a collection of about a dozen which we keep in a cool, dark place and bring out whenever we need to mix a special mind-potion for use in the bath. Our favourites are rosemary, lavender, sandalwood and camomile. Add essential oils to the water as the bath is filling, using about 10–15 drops total of either a single essence or of a mixture for a large bath. Let them work their wonders while you carry out a relaxing and waste-eliminating self-massage. When your bath is finished,

lie down for 10 minutes with an eye mask or a piece of dark fabric across your eyes and keep warm. It should leave you feeling like a new woman.

THE MASSAGE MESSAGE
Water is the perfect medium for self-massage. The heat of the water works silent wonders and it supports your body so that you have easy access to feet, legs, arms and torso while still remaining relaxed. When you get into the bath, gently scrub yourself all over with a hemp glove or a loofa (a dried vegetable relative of the cucumber). Then just relax and soak for a few minutes, letting the heat penetrate your muscles. Keep a cool cloth nearby to smooth over your face when needed.

Now you are ready for massage, which is nothing more than stroking, kneading, pushing and pressing your skin and muscles. Start with your feet. Grasp one foot between thumb and fingers and press in between the tendons, gently at first, then harder and harder, moving from the toes up towards the ankle. Then, using your fingertips and knuckles, go over the soles of your feet (see p. 39). Wherever you find a sore spot, work harder until you feel the discomfort melt beneath your hand. Now do your heel, grasping it between thumb and fingers and working around the area of the Achilles tendon. This is also a good time to make circles with your foot to loosen the ankle joint. Repeat this with the other foot and then go on to your legs.

Lift each leg in turn and deeply stroke the flesh on the back, from the ankle up to the knee. Then go back to the ankle again and repeat the same motions on the side and front of the calf. Keep working and, as you massage a little deeper with each stroke, you will gradually find that any tautness softens. Now go over your thighs with the same movement and afterwards knead and squeeze around the knee area wherever there are trouble spots, just as you did on the feet. Now knead each thigh and hip. Then go on to your arms.

Knead and squeeze every spot you can reach on your shoulders and neck, looking for sore spots and focussing on the areas between joints and muscles. Pay particular attention to the tops of shoulders, where most of us lock away our tension. Grasp this area in your thumb and fingers and insistently ease away any hardness you find there. Finally, go over your ribs, doing each side with its opposite hand, and then you are ready for the most relaxing movements of all: lymphatic drainage massage on your face and neck.

LYMPHATIC DRAINAGE MASSAGE
Lymphatic massage was taught to us by beauty therapist Eve Lom, a stunningly beautiful woman in her thirties whose hands literally work miracles in clearing away the debris which collects in the muscles of the face with fatigue. The whole routine takes about 10 minutes. To carry out pressure-release movements, you press firmly, slowly and rhythmically, then release, moving the fingertips across the skin's surface before pressing again in a new spot.

Cross your arms in front of you and lay your hands flat on your chest. Now in one smooth movement, slide your hands upwards to the neck and then draw them down over the chest until they are uncrossed, exerting firm but comfortable pressure on your skin. You can work first on one side and then on the other, or do both at once with the movement of one hand coming just behind the other. Repeat 10 times.

Now cross your arms, placing your right hand on your left elbow and vice versa. Slide your hands up along the arms and across the chest, with each hand finishing at the opposite armpit. Repeat 10 times.

Cross your arms and place your hands just behind your ears, using the right hand to massage the left side and the left hand for the right, moving your fingers down across your throat, all the while breathing deeply. Repeat 10 times.

Place your fingertips in the centre of your forehead and use a pressure-release gliding movement from the centre outwards towards the temple. Repeat 6 times.

Now firmly pinch your eyebrows with your thumbs and forefingers using a pressure-release movement from the inside outwards. Repeat 5 times.

To massage the sinus area, place the backs of your thumb-nails on either side of your nose at eye level. Using deep movements and a pressure-release glide, move the fingers outwards, towards the front of the ear. Then do the same movements under the cheeks and across the upper lip. Finish by carrying out a pinching movement with your thumbs and forefingers along the jaw line from the centre of the chin outwards.

This lymphatic drainage massage is also an important part of a detoxifying regime (see p. 121).

ESSENCE ALCHEMY
As part of the benevolent bath, choose essential oils not so much for what they can do for your skin as what they can do to expand your consciousness and lift your spirit. Whatever your negative state may be, it has an enchanting antidote from the world of flowers:

NEGATIVE STATE	ESSENTIAL OIL REMEDY
anger	ylang ylang, rose, camomile
resentment	rose
sadness	hyssop, marjoram, sandalwood
mental fatigue	basil, peppermint, cypress, patchouli
worry	lavender
feeling jaded	neroli, melissa, camphor
feelings of weakness	camomile, jasmine, melissa
irritability	frankincense, marjoram, lavender, camomile
physical exhaustion	jasmine, rosemary, juniper, patchouli
anxiety	sage, juniper, basil, jasmine

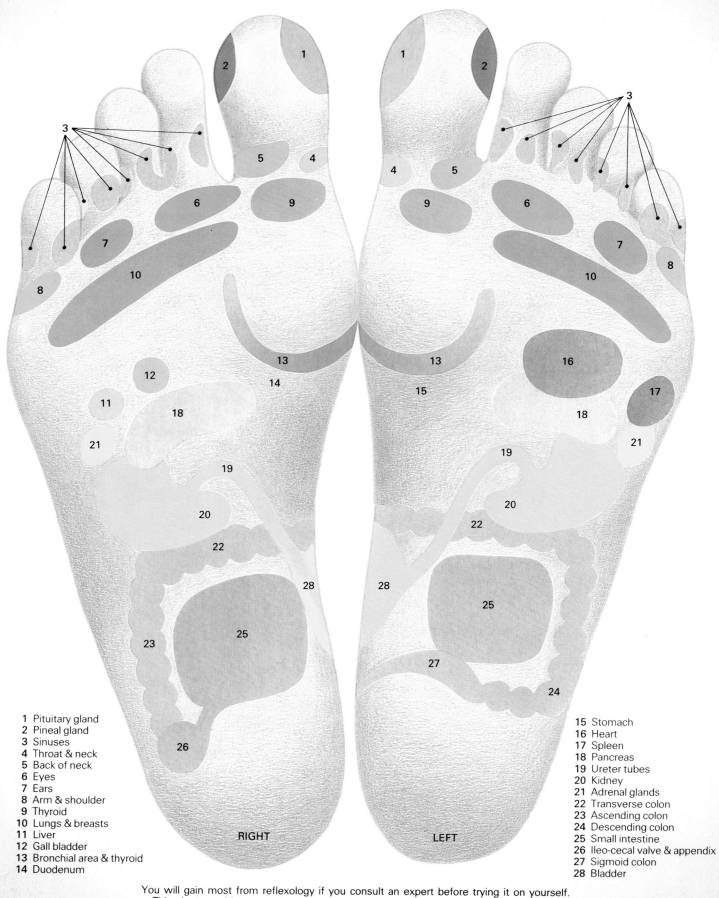

1 Pituitary gland
2 Pineal gland
3 Sinuses
4 Throat & neck
5 Back of neck
6 Eyes
7 Ears
8 Arm & shoulder
9 Thyroid
10 Lungs & breasts
11 Liver
12 Gall bladder
13 Bronchial area & thyroid
14 Duodenum

15 Stomach
16 Heart
17 Spleen
18 Pancreas
19 Ureter tubes
20 Kidney
21 Adrenal glands
22 Transverse colon
23 Ascending colon
24 Descending colon
25 Small intestine
26 Ileo-cecal valve & appendix
27 Sigmoid colon
28 Bladder

RIGHT   LEFT

You will gain most from reflexology if you consult an expert before trying it on yourself.
This chart provides general guidance – your own reflexology points may vary slightly.

to sleep so you'll be at your best in the morning . . . so what do you do?

Insomnia is incredibly frustrating because no matter how hard you *try* to sleep, it doesn't help. Fortunately, there are several first-aid techniques which, on their own or in combination, can help even the most confirmed insomniac to sleep.

● **Write your troubles away** If you can't sleep because your mind is racing, face all your thoughts rather than trying to block them from your head. Sit down with pen and paper, and write down all the things that come into your mind. Don't worry if you jump from one to another, just keep jotting down thoughts, ideas and worries. When you can think of no more to write, you can let go of all those concerns because they'll be right there on the paper when you wake up.

● **Hydro-help** There are two excellent hydrotherapy remedies for sleeplessness: the cold sitz bath and the wet socks treatment. Do one or the other immediately before you retire for the night.

For the sitz bath, fill a bath or a large basin with about five inches of cold water. Make sure you are warm and wear something to keep the upper half of your body warm. Lower your bottom into the water, but let your feet and legs hang over the edge of the bath or basin. Sit for 30–45 seconds, then get out and dry yourself. Wrap up warm and go to bed.

For the wet socks treatment, soak a pair of cotton socks in cold water, wring them out well and put them on. Cover them with a second pair of dry wool or cotton socks and retire for the night.

● **Relaxation exercise** A regular exercise, such as the Total Breath exercise, will go a long way towards making you more receptive to sleep. But if you're having real trouble unwinding, use a relaxation tape to guide you through the exercise to encourage relaxation for sleep. If possible, do the exercise in bed with a tape recorder close at hand which will switch itself off after you fall asleep. If your mind wanders away from the exercise at any point, don't worry. Gently bring your awareness back to the tape and continue.

● **Mellow music** Music, too, can help alter consciousness and have you sinking blissfully into the depths of slumber. Listening to your favourite soothing music in bed is one of the most pleasant ways of all to put a racing mind to rest and ease yourself into sleep. There

are also some wonderful 'New Age' tapes designed specifically for relaxation which incorporate soothing sounds, such as the ocean, together with harmonious instrumental sounds which still the mind and the body.

● **Sedative scents** Some of the essential plant oils have a wonderful calming effect on the mind and body. Take a warm bath, adding four drops of lavender oil, two drops of camomile oil and two drops of neroli (orange blossom) oil. Or place a drop or two of each on your pillow to inhale through the night.

NATURAL SLEEPING POTIONS

Sleeping pills are notoriously addictive and it is ultimately dangerous to rely on them as a means of knocking yourself out. Fortunately, there are some excellent natural alternatives.

● **Tryptophan** This free amino acid is a superb natural sedative which you can use either to help you get to sleep or just to calm you down when you need to unwind. Tryptophan works because it is used by your body to produce serotonin, a brain chemical important for relaxation and for inducing sleep. Many people, particularly as they get older, tend to have a deficiency of serotonin and suffer from the kind of nervousness which makes sleep difficult.

For a good send-off into blissful slumber, take 500–1000 mg of tryptophan together with a piece of fruit or wholemeal bread on an otherwise empty stomach about 30–45 minutes before bedtime. Tryptophan only works for relaxation if you can get it through the blood-brain barrier. The high-carbohydrate snack is therefore very important, since it encourages brain uptake of the free amino.

● **Passiflora pills** Passion flower, one of the world's best natural tranquillizers, is readily available in tablet form. Take them before going to bed or when you need a sedative to calm you down. Unlike tranquillizers, passiflora pills are not habit-forming. We take two to four tablets before going to bed when we need them.

● **Tranquillity teas** Two delicious herbal teas are recommended for relaxation: camomile and peppermint. Make them as you would an ordinary cup of tea and, if you like, sweeten with a teaspoon of honey. Another good bedtime drink is a tablespoon of orange flower water stirred into a cup of hot water and sweetened with a little honey.

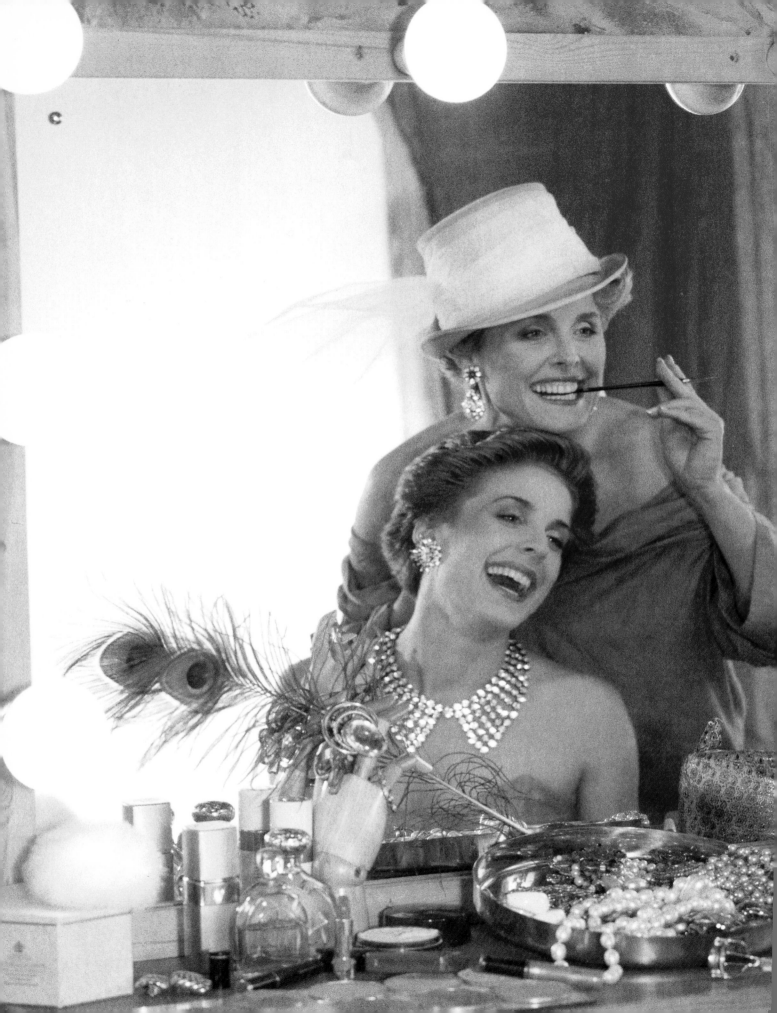

SHOW TIME

Take one handful of self-awareness, a generous portion of style, a spoonful of individuality and a pinch of wit. It's the archetypal recipe for glamour. And today's glamour is a whole new story.

That glamour is always changing is what gives it its power. The heavy-lidded made-up face of the 1930s spoke of opulence and lifted the imagination out of the grey, humdrum world into one filled with drama and seduction. Glamour in the 1950s was one of a different order – more girlish, coy, frilly and sexy – and without the same force. Then came flower power and ethnic dreams. In the 1960s and 1970s, when technology appeared a threat to human life, glamour called for home-spun beauty. Now it is different yet again, less showy and more fundamental, with its nearly naked face and wind-blown hair. Glamour now demands that you be yourself and express it. There is a new kind of boldness afoot. You see it in the surprising, fresh new colours used for make-up, in freer hairstyles and in a way of dressing that encourages you to mix unpredictable combinations, such as glittery earrings with faded jeans.

In some ways glamour is easier to achieve today because there is such emphasis on individuality. The notion of the 'perfect oval' face which women used to strive for is gone – we hope for good. If your face is square or your nose is large, let them be that way and be bold about it. They are great because they are a part of what makes you you. But in lots of ways new glamour is tougher too. Thirty years ago, when women wore hats with veils, and heavy black eye-liner, they could get away with skin that was less than perfect. And if your stomach wasn't flat or your waist wasn't waspish, there were always girdles.

In those days a woman remained under cover. Now there is no way you can hide neglect. That is why today's glamour begins from the *inside*, with a body that is strong and firm and vibrantly healthy, with eyes that shine and skin that glows, giving off a sustained radiance which comes from abundant energy. Today's glamour is hard work. It means eliminating from your life whatever is detrimental to you, such as coffee, cigarettes and excessive stress. It also means committing yourself to regularly practised relaxation or meditation, exercise and the very best diet you can manage. Only after this is it time for 'show time', the externals from first-rate skin care and looking after your teeth, nails, breasts and thighs to make-up and that most seductive of all areas of glamour – perfume.

But 'show time' is important. How you look matters. Not in some superficial or narcissistic way. It matters because the way you look is a reflection of how you feel about yourself and your life and how well you care for yourself. When you look good, you bring pleasure to those who know you – your partner, your children, friends and workmates. Also, unless you can care for yourself lovingly you will never be able wisely to care for others.

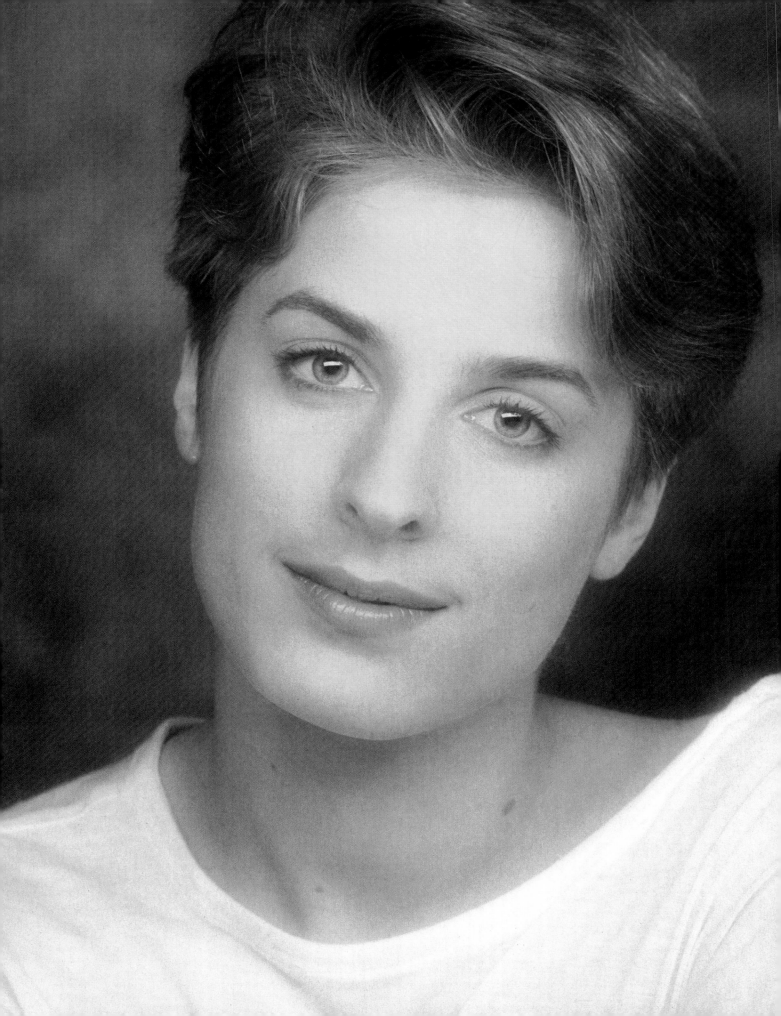

FACE THE DAY

Matt make-up can be magnificent – particularly in the daytime. It can make your face look elegant, clean, fresh and more beautiful than any other kind.

BUILD ON A GOOD FOUNDATION

The foundation, like the skin care products you choose, should be the very best you can afford. Choose a foundation which is just a shade darker than your basic skin tone. This will cover every little flaw on your face superbly. Make sure it is a flat beige or that it has a slightly yellow tone to it. Your colour should come from the blusher, not the foundation. The foundation is nothing more than a perfect canvas on which to work magic. It should look flat and perfect – not florid. Spread it on your well-moisturized skin with a very dry sponge, pressing it carefully and deeply into the skin.

POWDER PERFECT

Now is the time for powder (not necessarily at the end of your make-up, which is when most women usually apply it). Make sure you dust it on in every direction all over your face. Close your eyes and stretch the whole of the upper eye area while you powder it thoroughly so that the powder gets into every crevice. Then use a brush to brush any excess powder off in a downwards direction. Now examine any flaws still showing and correct them. This you can do with a tiny paint brush and the help of a cover-up cream or oil-based make-up stick in a toning shade.

THE EYES HAVE IT

Now brush your brows to get rid of excess powder and flaky skin. Then check to see if they need shaping. This needs to be done before you put even a hint of colour on your lids, for they create a frame within which to work and give you a defined area so you can get a sense of the shapes that are there and how best to work with colours to enhance them.

● **Matt shadows** Once the brow is done, apply the first of your matt eye-shadows. It needs to be a pale one – the palest you will use. *Off*-white is a good choice. It goes all over the eye area on which you intend to apply colour – from the eye's inner corner to the brow's outer edge and from eyelashes to brow. First press the colour into the skin with a sponge-tipped applicator and later blend with a brush. Next, apply the most prominent colour you are going to use. This will quickly give you a sense of what you are trying to achieve. Later you can apply your shader or highlighter. Remember that colours on the outer edges of your eyes will tend to widen the look of your face and open your gaze.

● **Bright eyes** You can give new life to tired eyes by colouring the underneath rim with a light-coloured pencil. This makes your eyes look bolder and more wide-awake. But it is not a technique you would use if your eyes are particularly prominent. Then a cool, dark colour inside the lid can bring glamour. One of a woman's most important accessories is an eyelash curler. It opens the eyes, makes you look bright and well, and is a wonderful pick-me-up. Ready for mascara. But what kind? Black or dark brown if your hair is dark. Redheads need a mink-grey or auburn mascara. Blondes need a brown or grey, and can even wear gold mascara if they like. Squeeze lashes gently for a few seconds with the curler, then apply mascara to both sides of your upper lashes.

BLUSH GENTLY

When it comes to blusher, go easy and go matt. Frosted blushers rarely look good. Apply it with a brush and never take it further in than the pupil of your eye.

LOVELY LIPS

Lips can shimmer if you like. Paint your mouth when it is closed, not open, using a brush in preference to a pencil, which can give too hard a line. A pencil can be useful, however, for a mouth that is too large because it makes it easy to create a new edge slightly inside the natural one. If your lips are too small, then put a dark outline on the outside and use a lighter lipstick within. If you apply gloss *never* put it all over your mouth or it will melt into the edges. Less is more. A little in the centre can give a perfect look to your mouth.

left **Susannah's matt make-up** for a natural daytime look.
Foundation: a flat neutral beige over the face;
Powder: a light dusting of a pale translucent shade;
Blusher: a warm peach powder blusher brushed liberally on cheekbones, browbones and chin for a natural glow;
Eyes: a bright blue crayon under eyes; matt apricot eye-shadow over the lids with a paler colour on the inner corner to open the eyes; brown mascara;
Lips: a warm peach shade.

Show Time

STEP INTO THE NIGHT

Frosted make-up can set your face alight. Sleek, shimmery, smooth skin that refracts the light gives an illusion of youth and fresh, glowing vitality as nothing else can – particularly in the middle of a grey winter. But shimmer is like fire. You've got to know how to use it or you'll get badly burned.

Make-up manufacturers have refined and developed the use of gold and silver fleck in foundations, lipsticks, cheek colours and eye-shadows to a peak of subtlety. The old-fashioned glitter is obvious, the new shimmer is anything but. Expertly applied it can look superb. Badly done it becomes a disaster. To turn base metal into gold (or silver for that matter), you've got to be an alchemist.

BRING OUT THE BEST
All frosted make-up draws attention to the part of your face on which you put it, so use it to accentuate your best features. This will help to detract from areas you don't want to make prominent. To get the best from shimmer – whether you're using a frosted foundation, lip colour, blusher or eye-shadow – alternate areas of your face which have matt finish and flat, neutral colours with other areas you've highlighted with shimmer. Put it on your ear-lobes, your bare shoulders, and on the sides of your neck, as well as on eyelids, cheeks, the tip of the chin and the mouth. But never wear a highly frosted lipstick if your lips are wrinkled. Instead, use matt lip colour and dab a spot of gold or platinum eye-shadow in the middle of the bottom lip.

PLAY DOWN IMPERFECTIONS
Some areas of the face should have no shine. Avoid drawing attention to any blemished or imperfect surface: under your eyes, between your nose and mouth and any wrinkled or lined part. And never put shimmer on your nose unless it is absolutely perfect. If it is, then you might draw a line of shimmer down the centre to draw attention to this fact.

HOW TO SHINE
When you make up an eye with shimmer, first use a flat, neutral colour for definition ... brown, mauve or grey. Then add your shimmer. But be careful to keep it away from the white of the eye or it will dull the natural sparkle in your eye. And always clear away any shimmer that has fallen on your cheeks before powdering.

GOLD OR SILVER?
If you look at a fine healthy skin, you'll find it has a natural, gold shimmer to it. Make-up containing minute gold flecks can be used to exaggerate this. Gold-frosted products give richness of tone and depth, make your face look more rounded, full-bodied and open. But you have to be very careful with them – it's tempting to get 'drunk' on gold.

Almost any woman can benefit from the warmth of make-up frosted with gold, but silver is special. It's reserved for the few who have perfect health and flawless skin. It calms the make-up, suits the cool colours in clothes for winter – deep blue, white or magenta – but it is less 'natural' than gold. And if you don't soften the cool sophisticated look of silver with a little warmth, for instance, by using pink and peach in the lip and cheek colours, it can either make you look weak and wan or cold and unapproachable. Silver shimmer is best used only at night. Try frosting high on your cheeks or at the bow of your lips before applying lipstick. Another place where silver shimmer works magic, even on its own, is at the inner corner of your eyes, where it makes them seem to sparkle.

These are basic rules, and of course rules are made to be broken. But go easy. It's better to use too little than too much.

right **Leslie's evening make-up** for a special occasion.
Foundation: a neutral cream concealer applied with a brush to cover dark circles under eyes and any flaws (carefully covered with fine translucent powder applied with a brush two minutes later); a warm foundation with a slight golden frost applied on a damp sponge for even tone;
Powder: a light coating of translucent powder in a similar shade to foundation applied across every area of the face – remove excess with a brush;

Blusher: peachy matt blusher for the outer cheeks, browbones, chin and forehead;
Eyes: defined with a matt neutral liner in charcoal above and below the eyes; matt pink eye-shadow and pale highlighting shadow on the browbones and inner corner of the lids to open out deep-set eyes; charcoal mascara carefully applied to top and lower lashes;
Lips: a deep pink shade for dramatic definition and highlighted with a dab of frosted eye-shadow in the centre of the lower lip.

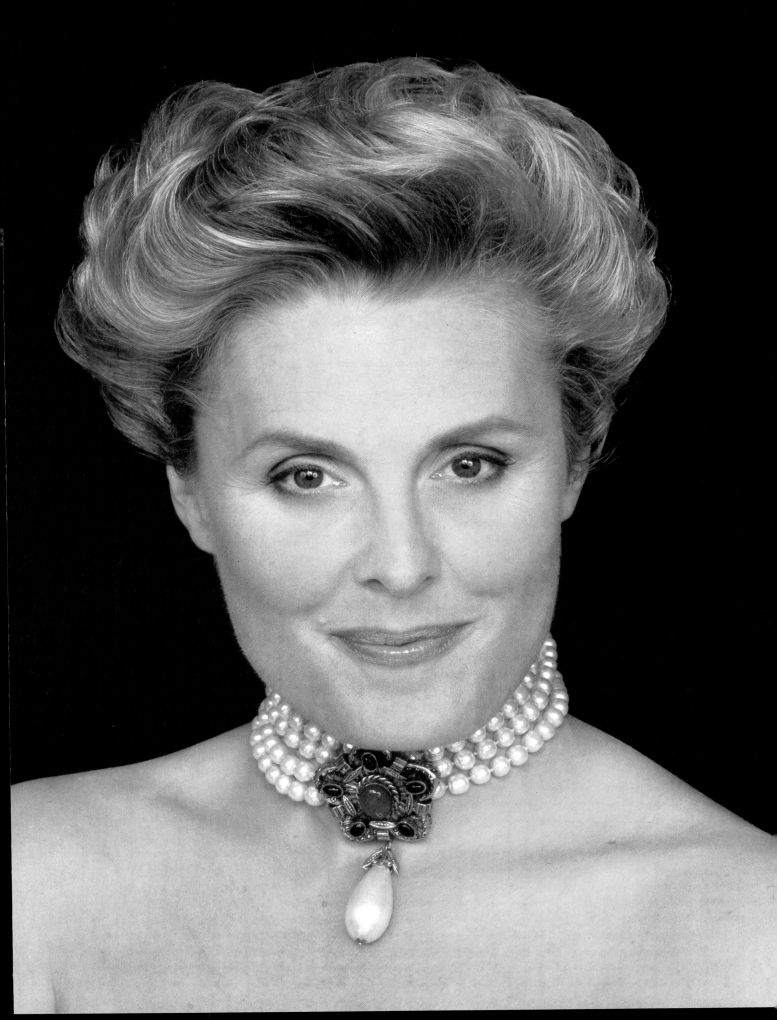

NAILS TO FLAUNT

Beautiful nails are no accident. A few fortunate women seem to have been born with genes which lend themselves to the growth of long, strong nails and healthy hair. The rest of us have to work at it. The encouraging thing is that a little work – some changes in nutrition plus a new regime of external care – can transform your nails within a few months. We know. We both used to belong to that group of women with nails like paper. Now they are strong and healthy and will grow just as long as we want to wear them.

WHY WEAK NAILS?
Your nails are made of keratin – a dehydrated tough protein similar to hair but considerably more mineralized. The standard advice (still, sadly, given by a lot of so-called nail experts) is that if your nails are weak or thin or break easily, you need to eat lots of protein to correct the condition. It is this assumption that leads manicurists to suggest gelatin capsules for weak nails. But it is a false one. Very soft nails, like flimsy or lifeless hair, most often announce not a protein deficiency, but either a mineral deficiency or a low level of hydrochloric acid and digestive enzymes in your body. This means that you are not able to break down the proteins in your food properly into their respective amino acids from which hormones, enzymes, muscle tissue, hair and (in this case) nails can be built.

The breakdown of proteins into amino acids which your body can use takes place in your digestive system thanks to the actions of hydrochloric acid and special enzymes. When insufficient hydrochloric acid is present in the stomach – something which is particularly common as people get older – then, even though you may be eating more than enough protein and even though you may be getting an ample supply of minerals such as calcium, magnesium, zinc, chromium and nickel from the foods you eat or from nutritional supplements you are taking, you still will not be absorbing them. The condition is a common one and it too often goes unrecognized. It is called hypochlorhydrin: lack of sufficient stomach acid.

Poor protein breakdown can also be the result of an insufficiency of proteolytic (protein-digesting) enzymes which tends to be a part of a vicious circle. Enzymes for breaking down proteins are made from amino acids, but if there are insufficient amino acids then you will not

have enough enzymes and therefore be even less able to break down proteins to make more. Without a good supply of digestive enzymes you will not be absorbing minerals adequately from your foods.

One of the best possible overall treatments for nails is to go on a six-week course of nutritional supplementation aimed at eliminating hypochlorhydrin, breaking through this vicious cycle and restoring normal digestion. This means taking three 500 mg capsules of a good blend of amino acids (ideally formulated to mimic the balance found naturally in an egg), together with one or two tablets of betaine hydrochloride and three to six kelp tablets after each meal. It is a method which tends to work even when all others fail. For anyone who has consistently struggled with the problem of poor nails it can be a real blessing.

NAIL GLAMOUR
Part of the fun of looking glamorous is having 10 beautiful lady-of-leisure nails to waft about. Yet who wants to spend their life wearing protective gloves and worrying about the 'catastrophe' of breaking a nail? Learn the French manicure secrets for strong nails and discover the nail-strengthening supplements. Then you can renew your manicure just once a week and take long, beautiful nails for granted.

● **Naked nails** As we've seen, like your hair and skin, your nails are an excellent reflection of your body's general state of health – and not only of the poor breakdown of protein in your digestive system. If you have always had a problem with growing your nails because they are weak or split easily, you should ask 'why?'. Too often, cosmetic companies which sell products to mask nail imperfections, such as a ridge-smoothing base coat, lead us to believe that if you have a particular nail problem it is normal and can't be helped. More often than not, nail problems are linked with dietary deficiencies. By discovering what these are you can get to the root of the problem and help yourself from the inside out.

● **External threats** Although many nail problems come from nutritional deficiencies, external factors such as detergents, chlorine in swimming pools, sun, wind and central heating can also contribute to damaged nails and chapped hands. It is best to wear rubber gloves to protect your hands when they have to be submerged in

COMMON PROBLEMS	REMEDY
Splitting/breaking nails Caused by deficiency in vitamin A and the sulphur amino acids.	Cod liver or halibut oil, liver, fresh carrot juice, egg yolks, cabbage and onions. Beta-carotene supplements for vitamin A (see p. 109).
Nail ridges Horizontal or vertical nail ridges usually indicate a B-complex vitamin deficiency.	Avoid refined flour and sugar and excess alcohol. Take a high-potency B-complex supplement. Blackstrap molasses, liver and whole grains are also high in B-complex vitamins.
Pale, thin dry nails Often due to a lack of iron.	Sun-dried raisins or apricots, leafy green vegetables, blackstrap molasses. Take iron supplements in conjunction with vitamin C and folic acid to aid absorption.
Hangnails Torn skin at base or side of nail indicates a lack of folic acid, vitamin C, essential fatty acids, or all three.	Evening primrose oil, folic acid and vitamin C supplements.
White spots and bands Not a calcium, but a zinc and B6 deficiency. (Particularly common in women who take the Pill.)	Zinc, B6 and B-complex supplements.

any sort of detergent or chemical solution. You can protect them against the elements by wearing a good barrier hand cream. This will help keep your natural skin moisture in and environmental pollutants out. Remember to use a sunscreen if your hands are exposed to ultraviolet sun rays for a period of time. Your hands, like your face, will show your age if neglected.

REPAIRS

If you do break a nail and can't bear the thought of cutting the other nine off, it is possible to repair it, although the process is long and frustrating. If you nick a nail you can fix it by applying a small amount of nail glue to the tear and then covering it with a couple of layers of clear polish. Be sure that the nail is not oily or the glue will not adhere. The best glue comes in a pen-like container which dispenses one fine drop at a time.

If you lose an entire nail tip, you can buy a pack of tips which you glue onto your own nail and then file down on the surface to smooth out the ridge. These tips are far better than the false nail horrors and less messy than the brush-on variety. Unfortunately, they are not as tenacious as your natural nails and you are likely to lose a tip to your rubber gloves.

NAIL-BITER'S HOPE

If you really are determined to break that old habit of biting your nails, first find a picture of a beautiful pair of hands with long nails in a magazine, cut it out and keep it in a prominent place for inspiration. Follow the Pre-Manicure (see p. 52) to tidy up your nails. Always keep polish on them and add an extra layer of top coat every day. Keep a nail file with you always and if you get a rough edge smooth it off immediately so that you won't be tempted to nibble it. Take pride in keeping your nails neat. Even very short nails can look attractive if they are well groomed and coated with clear polish. As your nails begin to grow, you can paint the tips white as described in the French Manicure. Pretty soon, with patience and care, you'll have nails to flaunt.

NAIL SAVER TIPS

Without becoming obsessive, there are certain precautions you can take to help protect your nails from physical damage:

● Use a pencil to dial the telephone.
● Use a knuckle rather than your fingertip to push buttons, for example to call a lift.
● Keep hand lotion ready to use after you wash your hands and during the day.
● Use rubber gloves *every* time you wash the dishes.

Show Time

51

THE FRENCH MANICURE

THE TOOLS
Nail varnish remover, cotton wool pads, emery board or emery file, nail soak (see 3 below), orange stick, cuticle trimmer, nail scissors, buffer (optional), base coat, nail varnish, top coat.

THE PRE-MANICURE
If you are short on time, just do steps 1 and 2. Save the longer pre-manicure for really pampering yourself.

1 Filing
It is best to file your nails while they still have polish on so that they are afforded some protection. Keep the sides of the nails straight and only file the corners in a gentle curve. Follow the natural shape of your nails as a guide. Never saw back and forth across the nails as this will cause them to split, but file away from the outer edge towards the centre in one direction.

2 Cleaning
Remove any varnish from nails with a nail varnish remover containing conditioner to help prevent drying out the nails. Soak a cotton pad with remover and press it onto the nail for a few seconds, then wipe it outwards away from the cuticle. If you have been wearing coloured varnish you may need to soak a cotton bud with remover and go around the edge of the cuticle to help lift away any remaining colour. If your nails are stained, use a cut piece of lemon to help dissolve the stain and whiten them.

3 Soaking
Soak your fingertips in a bowl of warm water containing a conditioning nail soak. You can make your own using a few drops of your favourite bath oil dissolved in water, or simply a tablespoon of vegetable oil in water.

4 Cuticle care
Rinse your hands and pat them dry. Using an orange stick, gently push back your cuticles. This will make your nails appear longer. If you have any hangnails, trim them with a cuticle trimmer, but avoid cutting back your cuticles this way as this will only make them grow back heavier and encourage hangnails.

5 Top abrasion
This step can be helpful if your nails have bad ridges while you are waiting for the nutritional supplements to affect the new nail growth. Also, if you do not like to wear nail varnish, you can get a polished look naturally. Using a special flexible buffing board with three different grades of roughness on it, simply buff the nail in one direction several times. Start with the heaviest grade and work towards the finest, which will leave your nails smooth and shining and less likely to flake and split. This also encourages blood flow to the cuticles and creates a smooth surface for your base coat to adhere to. But never overdo it.

6 Final squeak
Rub over each nail once more with a cotton pad soaked in nail varnish remover to prepare an oil-free base on which to apply your varnish.

THE MANICURE
Three steps to success:

1 The base
Apply a layer of protective base coat to each nail. Look for a base coat which incorporates nail strengthener.

2 Tip treat
Paint the tip of each nail – the white part – with white enamel. This can be matt white or pearlized white. This is a great improvement on the old-fashioned nail pencil under the tip. Not only does it keep your nails looking fresh and clean but, more importantly, it gives them extra strength at the tips where they need it. Let the tips dry and then add another tip coat.

3 Top
Finish the manicure by applying a layer of top coat to the entire nail to seal the lacquers. You can also paint a little top coat under the tip of each nail for added protection. To keep your manicure fresh and protect your nails even further, paint a coat of top coat over the top of your manicure every evening and massage a little cuticle cream into your cuticles.

You can adapt the French Manicure for coloured nail varnish by using base coat in the same way and applying a layer of the coloured lacquer to the tips and allowing it to dry before adding two more coats of coloured polish to the entire nail and finishing with top coat. If you are using a darker colour, always paint the strokes lengthwise beginning with a centre stroke, and then paint either side. Do not take the polish quite to the edges of the nail sides. This will give your nails a longer, slimmer look and avoid staining your cuticles.

MANICURE TIPS
○ Be sure to allow each coat of polish to dry before applying the next. It is time-consuming, but it saves smudging a nail and starting all over again.

○ If you suffer from extreme impatience, invest in some quick nail enamel drier. The spray-on type is best and can cut down considerably on the time of your manicure.

○ Make sure you wipe the tops of your bottles of nail polish clean with a tissue before closing them tightly. This will help keep the polish from going thick and gooey.

○ If your polish does get thick, use some nail enamel solvent to thin it – thick polish takes even longer to dry.

right **The French Manicure** leaves your nails beautifully groomed but with a natural appearance that suits any type of clothes or make-up.

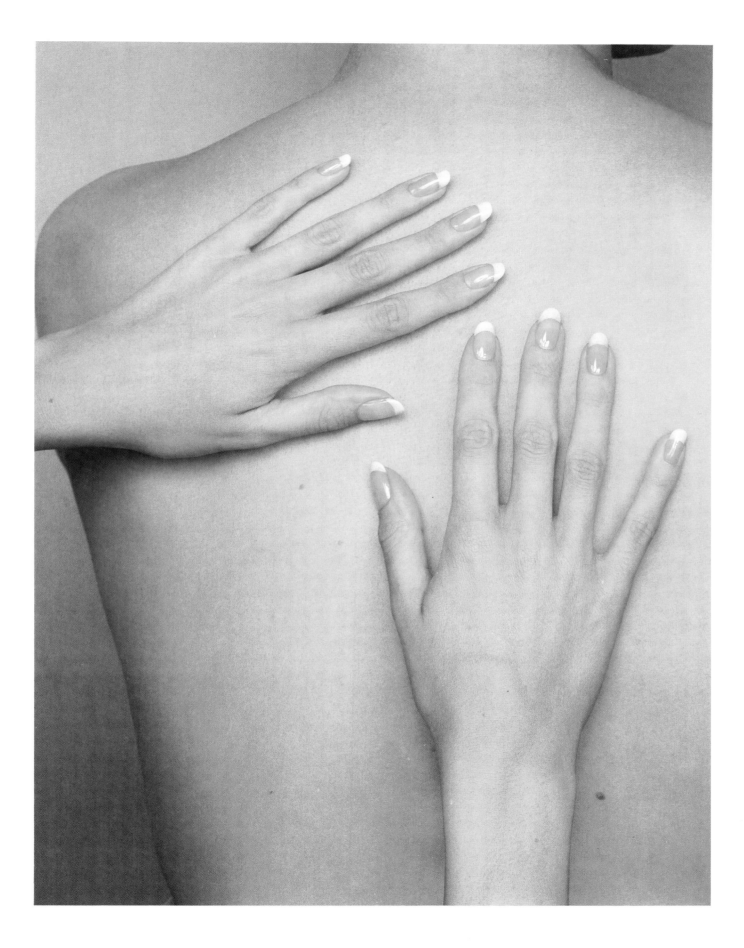

THE SEDUCTIVE SMILE

Teeth are boring. Everybody knows that. They are the part of the body most of us least like to concern ourselves with. For there is no glamour to be had from toothbrushes and dental floss. Or is there? In fact, your teeth are one of your most important assets for looking good. A number of classic studies where people are asked to look at photographs of faces and rate them according to attractiveness show that the single most determining criterion of attractiveness is not eyes, the shape of the face or the hair, but the teeth.

A staggering proportion of well-educated, well-heeled, and otherwise aware people are almost completely ignorant of how to look after their teeth and of how important the set of their jaw is to the way they look and feel. Dealing with diseases of the mouth has traditionally been considered almost entirely a matter of carrying out different mechanical procedures, such as fillings, crowns, bridges and root canal work, without any consideration of how this work might be affecting an individual's overall mental and physical health nor of how his overall dietary patterns and life style might be affecting the state of his teeth, mouth and jaw.

There are also a number of common fantasies about teeth which have no basis in fact. For instance, most people believe that tooth loss is a normal part of the aging process. Far from it. Although the vast majority of people over 60 no longer have their teeth, this, like other degenerative diseases, is nothing more than a pathological condition – the result of poor dental hygiene and of a nutritional life style which does not encourage high-level health. There is nothing whatever normal about it. People of non-Westernized cultures who live largely on diets of unrefined foods not only do not lose teeth, they also show no signs of either tooth decay or gum disease. And these peoples have never even heard of a dentist.

Another common 'tooth fairy' myth is the notion that tooth decay is the major cause of tooth loss. This is simply untrue. The average person has only six to ten teeth destroyed as a result of dental cavities. The remainder are lost through gum disease, called pyorrhoea or peridontal disease. It is something you need to know about to look after your seductive smile.

● **Peridontal disease** This is quite different from tooth decay. Instead of attacking the teeth themselves, it hits their support systems. It begins with an inflammation of the gums, then spreads to the ligaments and bones which are responsible for holding the teeth firmly in the jaw. Slowly and insidiously, it weakens this support system so that the teeth fall out. Gum disease is easy to spot. It goes through two stages. Symptoms of the first stage (called mild gingivitis) are simple: redness and swelling of the gums, as well as bleeding when you use dental floss. The second stage (peridontis) usually begins to manifest slowly but with alarming symptoms: severe redness and gum swelling, chronic bad breath, receding gums, gum bleeding even from gentle stimulation (say, when you are brushing your teeth), a build-up of calculus or tartar at the gumline and a feeling that your teeth are loosening from their sockets.

If you develop any of these symptoms, you should consult a dentist immediately – but one who is strongly oriented towards prevention. If teeth are already loose, everything possible (and that's a lot) should be done to tighten them before the word 'extraction' is even spoken. Far too many dentists are quick to drill or pull teeth which, with proper daily care and nutritional support, could be saved. And the loss of even one tooth is a serious business.

Research shows that oral contraceptives, emotional stress and smoking all reduce your body's defence against gum disease. So does a less-than-adequate diet, particularly any deficiency of calcium, magnesium or zinc. (There are also indications that supplements of these three minerals can dramatically improve the health of teeth and gums in some people.)

STRONG GUMS AND FIRM TEETH
As with tooth decay, the real answer to gum disease lies in *prevention* and in day-to-day treatment, as well as in support from your dentist or hygienist in eliminating that dark villain of teeth destruction: plaque. A sticky transparent film made up of bacteria and decomposed food particles, plaque is the number one cause of peridontal disease. It builds up on the surface of teeth and gets lodged into areas of the teeth which are hard to reach – for instance, in the spaces and crevices between the teeth at the gumline. If plaque is not cleared away within 24–36 hours it begins to harden into calculus, a deposit of hard calcium salts.

Plaque bacteria love sugar and refined carbohydrates, such as pasta, white bread and most breakfast cereals.

They hate raw fibrous fruits and vegetables, such as carrots, celery and apples. These and most other fresh raw foods act as natural cleansing agents.

● **How to remove plaque** It is not enough to stand in front of the bathroom mirror twice a day scrubbing back and forth with whatever toothbrush happens to be at hand. A hard- or medium-bristled toothbrush is more likely to scrape your gums from your teeth than remove plaque. The real challenge anyway is not removing plaque from teeth surfaces – that's easy – but rather from the spaces between the teeth and between the teeth and gums. For this you need a small soft brush with thin flexible nylon bristles (arranged in a straight line) which have been rounded off and polished so that the tip of each filament does not dig into or scrape away tooth or gum tissue.

Place the bristles of your soft brush into the crevice where teeth and gums meet and push them in as far as they will go at an angle of about 45 degrees to the length of the tooth. Now firmly wriggle the brush back and forth with small, almost circular strokes for a few seconds to dislodge plaque from the tooth; then whisk the brush upwards (or downwards if you are doing the top teeth) to the tooth's edge. Move on to the next tooth, proceeding in the same way. To clean the inside surfaces of your teeth, follow the same method. To brush the biting surfaces, put the bristles on top of each tooth, pressing firmly, and vibrate the brush back and forth with tiny strokes. When first using this method, your gums may bleed. If they do, it means either that your toothbrush is too hard or that they are unhealthy.

● **Make your own toothpaste** What about toothpaste? It is *not* essential for removing plaque. Brushing is. In most cases the only help it offers lies in its foaming action. In some cases toothpastes can be actively harmful, particularly those containing a high level of abrasives. You can do just as well with baking soda or salt or nothing at all.

● **Flossed perfection** Flossing gently scrapes the plaque away between each tooth and under the gums and it is essential that it is done at least once a day to prevent and alleviate gum problems.

Take a 2 foot (.6 m) strand of dental floss (waxed or unwaxed, as you prefer) and wind it around your middle fingers. Now, grasping the floss firmly between your thumbs and forefingers, gently ease it through the contact areas between each tooth and down as far as it will go between tooth and gum. Pressing the floss firmly against the tooth, scrape it up and down several times. As it becomes frayed, wind it around one finger another time so you have a new part of the floss to work with. Now loop the floss into a C-curve and gently scrape each tooth under the gums. To check on your progress with brushing and flossing, chew a 'disclosing tablet' before and after each brushing session in the beginning. Then, once you get the hang of it all, chew one once a week to check up on efficacy.

● **Quick help for gums** If you find your gums bleeding or you show any other signs of gum weakness, try rinsing your mouth with two solutions. First, mix a little hydrogen peroxide with equal amounts of water (as hot as you can stand it), slosh it around your mouth for half a minute, then spit it out. This will penetrate deep into any infected area, killing bacteria and transporting necessary oxygen to cells which have been damaged. Then wait 5 minutes and rinse again with a solution of half a teaspoon of salt in a glass of water. This helps shrink gums. You can go through this rinsing routine three times a day until bleeding subsides and then cut down to only once a day.

● **Cosmetic help for teeth** Good cosmetic treatment can transform the look of a face. But in order to bring lasting aesthetic results, any cosmetic treatment – large or small – has to be built on strong foundations.

Much crown and bridge cosmetic work is done without regard to its effect on the bite. And the great bulk of cosmetic dentistry is constructed not on a proper articulator which will reproduce all the sophisticated range of movements your jaw can make, but on a hinge articulator whose movements are far too limited. Crown and bridge work done this way – without regard to the occlusion functions or in the mouth of someone not carrying out good oral hygiene day after day – will invariably cause problems. Cosmetic work is nothing more than super precision work where crowns are made to fit accurately at the gum margin and all the crown and bridge work is made with as careful a regard for its being in harmony with the occlusion as for its cosmetic purposes. It sounds deceptively simple, but don't be fooled. Like everything else involved with maintaining beautiful, strong and healthy teeth and gums, there is far more to it than meets the eye.

SINGULAR SCENTSATIONS

The most potent beauty messages that you will ever send out come from the scent you wear. There are several thousand natural and man-made odorous materials that go into making perfumes. Each has its own special quality and many have specific effects on mind and body. Until this century, these were almost entirely taken from plants and flowers, with the exception of a few remarkable animal substances, like musk from the Tibetan deer, civet from the glands of the Abyssinian cat and ambergris from the sperm whale. This century, chemists have developed a wide variety of synthetic materials called aromatics which have new smells, quite different from natural oils. Some of our finest modern scents rely heavily on them.

MAKE FRIENDS WITH THE FAMILIES

Scents fall roughly into four families – floral, Oriental, green and aldehydic. Building a good scent 'wardrobe' depends on choosing one or two that you like best from each category and then experimenting with them. This needn't be as expensive as it sounds – particularly if you buy your perfumes duty-free. Also, thanks to improved synthetics, some of the new lower- and middle-priced scents are hard to beat. They may be cheap, but they certainly don't smell it. Of course, you will get a more elaborately constructed, longer lasting scent if you choose from the higher price range, because a good expensive scent develops on the skin, gradually unfolding its full perfume to give a sense of lasting luxury. But the less expensive scents, like Cacharel's Anaïs Anaïs, Elizabeth Arden's Blue Grass and Revlon's Jontue, challenge their higher-priced competitors for style.

⬤ **The feminine florals** Made from fragrant blossoms, the floral scents rely heavily on jasmine, tuberose, rose, lily of the valley and gardenia. Florals are feminine and easy to wear. The simple florals are pure fantasy and charming, never heavy, always womanly. You can wear them anywhere at any time. They are the hallmark of women who like the idea of being feminine and have no wish to hide it. Classics include Fidgi by Guy Laroche, Joy by Jean Patou, the elegant First by Van Cleef & Arpels, Nina Ricci's delicate L'Air du Temps, Revlon's Charlie, Oscar de la Renta, Lagerfeld's inimitable Chloé, Guerlain's fantasy fragrance Jardins de Bagatelle, Diorissimo and Poison from Christian Dior and the fabulous Diva by Ungaro.

⬤ **The mysterious Orientals** Oriental perfumes are full-blooded, sultry scents made from rich Eastern woods and grasses. Overtly seductive, they often include the nostalgic odour of vanilla or are tempered by more than a hint of spice. Women who prefer the Orientals like to be noticed. Wear them when you're feeling your most bold. This doesn't mean they have to be confined to slinky black dresses; they're great with jeans too. The traditional Oriental scents include Estée Lauder's Youth Dew and Cinnabar, Guerlain's Shalimar, Bal à Versailles and Scheherazade by Jean Desprez, Dioressence by Dior, Lancôme's dark and mysterious Magie Noire, Yves St Laurent's Opium and Calvin Klein's totally seductive Obsession.

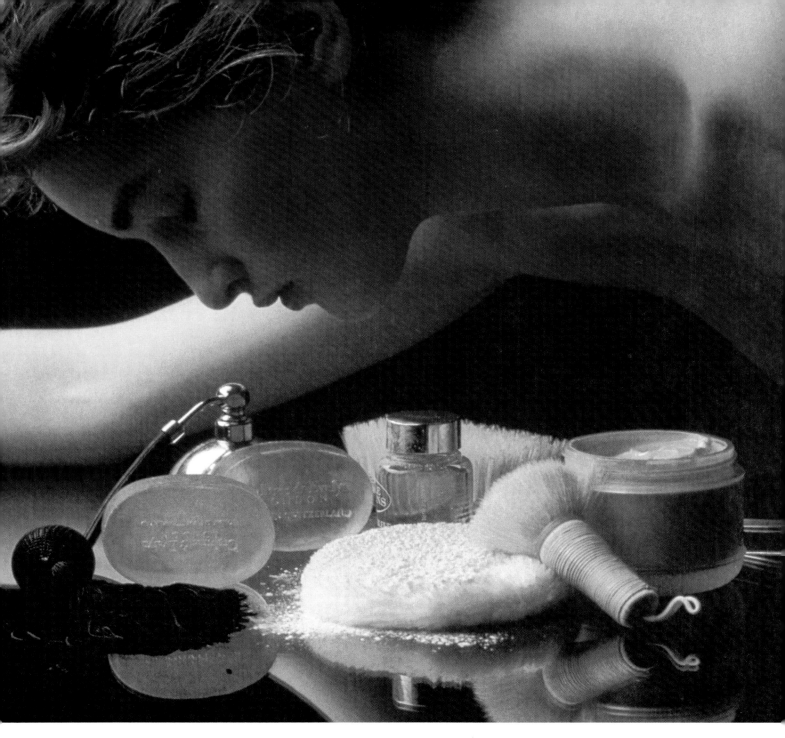

● **Cool greens** These scents are cool and biting, crisp and dry. Perfect for early mornings and when you feel so confident that you need only a light perfume to express your exuberance. This family of fragrances usually appeals to women who prize their independence and freedom, who like to think of themselves as moving swiftly and thinking clearly. The greens are dynamic, clear and never cloying, as some of the heavier perfumes can be. They rely on aromatic woods like cedar and sandalwood, mosses, ferns and grasses for their unique character. The classic greens include Balmain's Vent Vert, Yves St Laurent's 'Y', Estée Lauder's Alliage and Private Collection, Chanel No. 19, Balmain's lovely Ivoire and Givenchy III.

● **Aldehydics – scents for the city** The sophisticated 'moderns' are the aldehydics. Chanel No. 5 was the first in the family. Based on aldehydes – chemical substances with an obtrusive smell that gives an unmistakable power to any perfume – they are characterized by a rich, floral quality usually based on citrus, jasmine, rose and geranium plus musk. They can be worn by anyone but they belong to the city, with all its cultural and intellectual excitement. The classics include Arpège by Lanvin, Nina Ricci's Farouche, Calandre by Paco Rabanne, Guerlain's Chamade and Nahéma, Hermès' charming Calèche, Estée Lauder's White Linen, Molyneux's Vivre, Yves St Laurent's Rive Gauche, Mystère by Rochas, Carven's Ma Griffe and Givenchy's L'Interdit.

Show Time

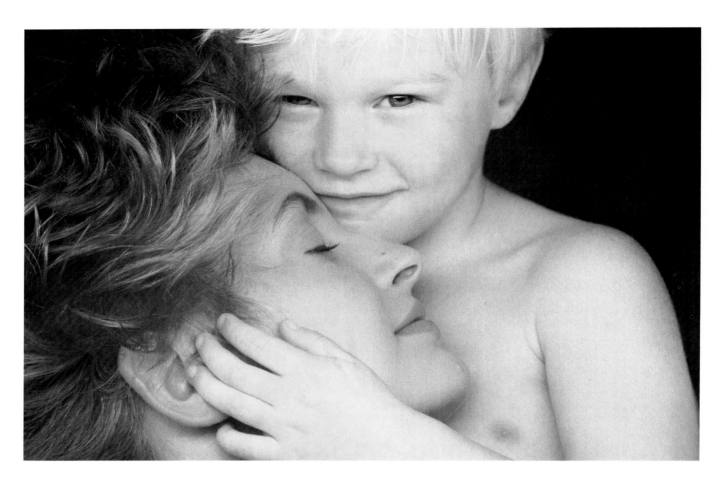

SATIN SKIN

To have good skin you need to look after it. There are two ways – the Bare Essentials and the Full Treatment. Which you choose depends on your age, your life style and the state of your wallet. For years both of us have followed the Bare Essentials with very good results. Recently, however, we have been experimenting with the Full Treatment, which was taught to us by Arsho Grimwood, one of the world's most accomplished beauty therapists and a woman with skin that looks 20 years younger than she is. We have been surprised to learn how much it has improved the texture and look of our skin – skin which was already good in the first place.

SAVE YOUR SKIN

Until now, cleansing, moisturizing and protecting our skin from ultraviolet damage was about as much as either of us felt we could manage. Otherwise, we believed, it would simply get too time-consuming and there were more interesting things to do than sit in front of a mirror messing about with skin preparations. But experimenting with Arsho's regime has changed our thinking. We have found that advanced skin care can easily be sandwiched in with other things in our daily routines and need not consume extra time.

For instance, we'd never used a mask. Then we tried wearing one while we are exercising in the morning. We simply put it on and head out the door for a run. The improved circulation and the open pores which come from an aerobic activity create a condition in which your skin is more receptive than it is at any other time to whatever you put on it. Why not use that opportunity to put on a deep moisturizing formula, an ampoule treatment, a mask or simply some vitamin A, which you can tissue off or wash away while you are in the shower? It is like getting all the benefits of a salon treatment with none of the time wasted and little of the hassle. We keep a drawer full of various goodies to use in this way – masks, sweet almond or sesame oil, vitamins E and A and evening primrose capsules and ampoules.

Apart from the basics of cleansing, moisturizing and protecting, the major prerequisite of any effective skin care programme is that you regularly change the treatment products or substances you are using on your face. We never use a single treatment product for more than two weeks at a time. Doing this means that you are always getting the most out of what you are using. Every tradition of natural health and beauty insists on this kind of change so that your system does not adapt itself to the active ingredients and stop being stimulated by them.

Here, briefly, are the outlines for both systems. Choose whatever is best for you. But if you choose the Bare Essentials, set it aside for a couple of weeks in spring and autumn each year and go for the Full Treatment. You'll be pleased at what it can do for you.

A SPOT OF HELP

Over the years we have experimented with dozens of home remedies for the occasional (or not so occasional) spot or pimple. Some of the things we've tried have been pretty bizarre – like the time Leslie decided to clear up a tiny pimple using crushed garlic because she had a photo session in three days' time and didn't want it to show. (She has a tendency toward excessive enthusiasm – and this was a case in point.) Her basic idea was sound. Garlic does indeed have anti-bacterial properties and has been used in folk medicine to draw out impurities in wounds and promote more rapid healing. But she did rather overdo it this time. Instead of a tiny speck of garlic pressed carefully for a short time over the little blemish, she crushed a whole clove, put it onto a plaster bandage and applied that to her face.

It worked, the spot cleared up almost immediately. The only trouble was, in the process she burned a hole in her skin almost two inches (5 cm) in diameter. The photography session had to be cancelled and she walked around for the next two weeks looking like either she had some rare form of degenerative skin disease or she had been beaten up rather badly. Since then she has steered clear of garlic as a cure for spots.

What we *do* use, and very successfully, is 1 teaspoon of ascorbic acid (vitamin C) powder dissolved in 4 fl oz (½ cup/112 ml) of water. We keep it in the bathroom in a little jar and apply a drop or two at once to any skin troubles which start to develop. It is a real wonder-worker. You can use the same mixture for about a month, then you need to mix up some more, for it does gradually lose its potency. It is the cheapest and most effective spot remover we've ever discovered.

SKIN CARE

THE BARE ESSENTIALS

Morning
○ Cleanse skin thoroughly with a toner or a little soap and water. Or use a cleansing facial scrub.
○ Moisturize with a product containing essential fatty acids (particularly if your skin is dry) and a sunscreen.
○ Apply a strong sunscreen in summer if you are going to be outside exercising or exposed to strong sunlight for a long period.

Evening
○ Cleanse your skin first with a lotion or cream cleanser and then with a wash-off cleanser to remove every trace of make-up and all the by-products of polluted air.
○ Use a toner if you wish, but it is not absolutely necessary.
○ Apply a good moisturizer or night cream.

THE FULL TREATMENT

On rising
○ Cleanse skin thoroughly with a toner on cotton pads until they come clean.
○ Apply either a mask, an ampoule, a treatment oil or vitamins which have been squeezed from a capsule pierced with a pin.
○ Leave on for at least 10, preferably 20, minutes while you bathe or exercise. (Or for as long as you like if you are exercising.) Be sure to change the treatment you are using every few days.
○ Remove all traces of this with a toner or soap and water as you bathe or shower.
○ Apply an eye cream to the eye area, a throat cream to the neck and a moisturizer with a sunscreen in it.
○ Remember to use an extra-strong sunscreen when you are outdoors in summer or exercising in the sun.

Late afternoon/early evening
○ Remove any make-up or grime using first a cream or lotion and then a wash-off cleanser, following with a toner if you like.
○ Now apply an ampoule of treatment oil. If you have time, steam your face over a basin of boiled water for a few minutes, using a towel over your head to concentrate the steam. This will open up your pores and help them drink up the oil. Leave the treatment on for 20 minutes (or for the evening if you are going to be at home or not going to wear make-up), then remove it with a little toner on a cotton pad and apply evening make-up if you want to wear it. (We often wear none. You'd be surprised, once your skin is in really top condition, how little you need to feel good enough to go out with a naked face.)

Before bed
○ Remove all make-up as above if you are wearing it. If not, use some toner on a cotton pad to wipe down your face.
○ Apply your night cream. And be sure to change it every fortnight. (If you have two or three, you can alternate, going from one to the next every two weeks, so this is no more expensive than using a single night cream as most women do.)

HAPPY HAIR

You could learn a lot about hair care from your vet. As every vet knows, the condition of an animal's coat depends more than anything else on its diet. If your dog starts to moult excessively or his coat loses its sheen or its colour, the vet will take a good look at what the animal is eating and decide whether it needs any special supplements added to its diet. Yet the connection between proper nutrition and a good healthy head of human hair is still often ignored. The same that can be said for the effect of inadequate breakdown of protein in the digestive system on nails can be said of poor hair (see p. 50). And the same free amino acid formula, together with betaine hydrochloride and kelp (plus a good B-complex formula – see below), can be a tremendous technique for restoring strength, body and shine to a head of hair which has lost it.

THE HAIR-MAKERS

Two free amino acids are particularly important for strong, healthy hair: cysteine and methionine. They are the sulphur-based aminos out of which your hair's protein – the keratin – is largely built. Cysteine is not an essential amino acid in the sense that it can be made in your body from methionine. But this conversion involves two vitamins – folic acid and B12 – neither of which are always in good supply, particularly among people who have lived on the typical Western diet high in sugar, alcohol and refined carbohydrates. Taking the free amino acid cysteine together with methionine and the co-factor nutrients helps bring about a rapid improvement in the look and feel of hair. Sometimes even within a few days you can notice a difference.

But protein is only the beginning of the healthy hair story. For in order to make proper use of it you have to have sufficient enzymes, a great many of which depend on there being enough zinc in your body. That's why a low level of zinc is a prime contributor to poor hair and one of the main reasons why women on the Pill and pregnant women often have hair in bad condition. Increased oestrogen levels often lead to falling zinc levels. When this occurs both hair and skin suffer. And, because of the overall effects of insufficient zinc on a woman's mental and physical health, more and more doctors are recommending nutritional supplements of zinc plus the nutrients to which its actions in the body are related – B2, B6, B12, folic acid and vitamin C – for

Pill-takers and mothers-to-be. When these supplements are given to women with hair problems, the problems often dramatically disappear.

Probably the most important of all the nutrients as far as the health and appearance of your hair are concerned are the B-complex vitamins. Research has shown that deficiencies of vitamins such as riboflavin, PABA, biotin, inositol, B6 and pantothenic acid (along with vitamin E) impair hair growth. The best sources of the B vitamins are brewer's yeast, liver, wholegrain cereals and breads, and blackstrap molasses. You can eat liver several times a week or stir a teaspoon of brewer's yeast into a glass of fruit juice a couple of times a day. Sugar, alcohol and caffeine destroy the B vitamins in your body and are among the worst things you can consume if you want your hair to stay healthy and beautiful.

Two trace elements – sulphur and iodine – are also high on the list of beautiful hair encouragers. Sulphur works closely with some of the B vitamins to keep hair strong and glossy. One of the reasons why many women get less than optimum quantities of sulphur in their diet is that they avoid eating eggs. Six to eight eggs a week can do wonders for a head of neglected hair, provided the rest of your diet is adequate as well. Oriental women traditionally keep their hair lustrous by adding seaweed (the best nutritional source of iodine you can find) to their dishes. Alternatively, you can take dried kelp tablets – one of the most remarkable internal treatments for hair you'll find anywhere.

Of course, all these nutritional aids must be combined with a good healthy diet if they are to work their wonders – a diet which stresses natural, unprocessed foods, is low in fat and sugar and high in fresh vegetables and fruits, as well as lean, good-quality proteins.

A CUT ABOVE THE REST

Hair, no matter how shiny and strong, needs to be cut well. You want to find the very best haircutter you can and hold on to him or her. A good cut can make you look and feel great, no matter what length your hair and no matter what your age. We keep our hair short. This is not because we adore short hair, but rather because we exercise a lot and, since both of us have very thick hair, it takes far too long to wash and dry it every day if it is longer than a few inches. If you are one of the lucky few

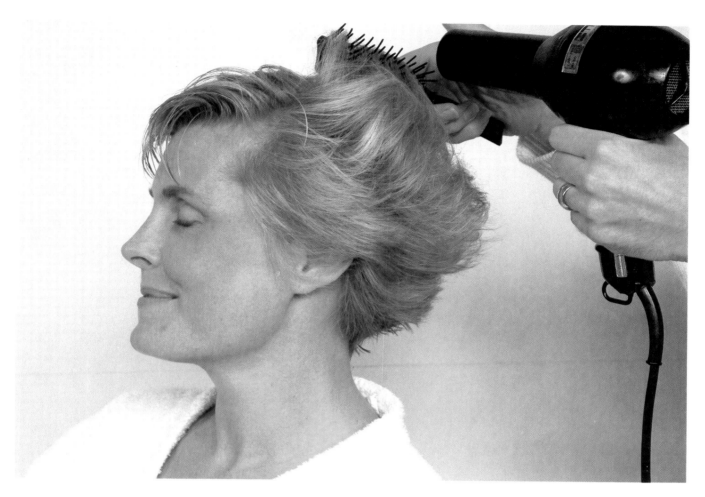

who can exercise vigorously without ending up in a pool of sweat then you can get away with long luxurious hair. We are not so lucky. Whatever hairstyle you do choose, it needs to fit in with your life style. Are you willing every day to spend 20 minutes doing it? Do you have time? How do you like to look? Simple and stylish? Soft and feminine? Glamorous? All of these things need to be taken into consideration when deciding how to have your hair cut.

Colour? Yes, if you can afford to and if you don't mind the fuss. But have it done professionally. Even so, it can become a terrible chore to look after – having to go to the colourist every six weeks to have roots redone. One way round this is to have gentle highlights done, where very small portions of hair are bleached and the rest is left natural. This, too, needs to be done professionally. But it can be relatively easy because it doesn't have to be redone more than approximately three times a year.

Finding the right shampoo and conditioner (if you use one) for you is very much dependent upon a lot of trial and error. What works for you will not necessarily work for a friend, even if she appears to have the same kind of hair you have. For us, how often we shampoo depends entirely on how often we exercise stren-

uously. And since that is usually six or seven times a week, we tend to wash our hair daily. Such frequent washing demands a gentle shampoo which does not strip the hair of natural oils and does not dry the scalp.

HAIR HELP
A good nutritional formula for strengthening hair would look something like this. These quantities would be taken three times a day with meals:

Kelp	6 tablets
Vitamin B1	15 mg
Vitamin B2	50 mg
Vitamin B3	25 mg
Pantothenic acid	250 mg
Vitamin B6	30 mg
Biotin	1000 mcg
Folic acid	400 mcg
PABA	50 mg
Choline	250 mg
Inositol	250 mg
Zinc	10 mg
L-cysteine	250 mg
L-methionine	250 mg

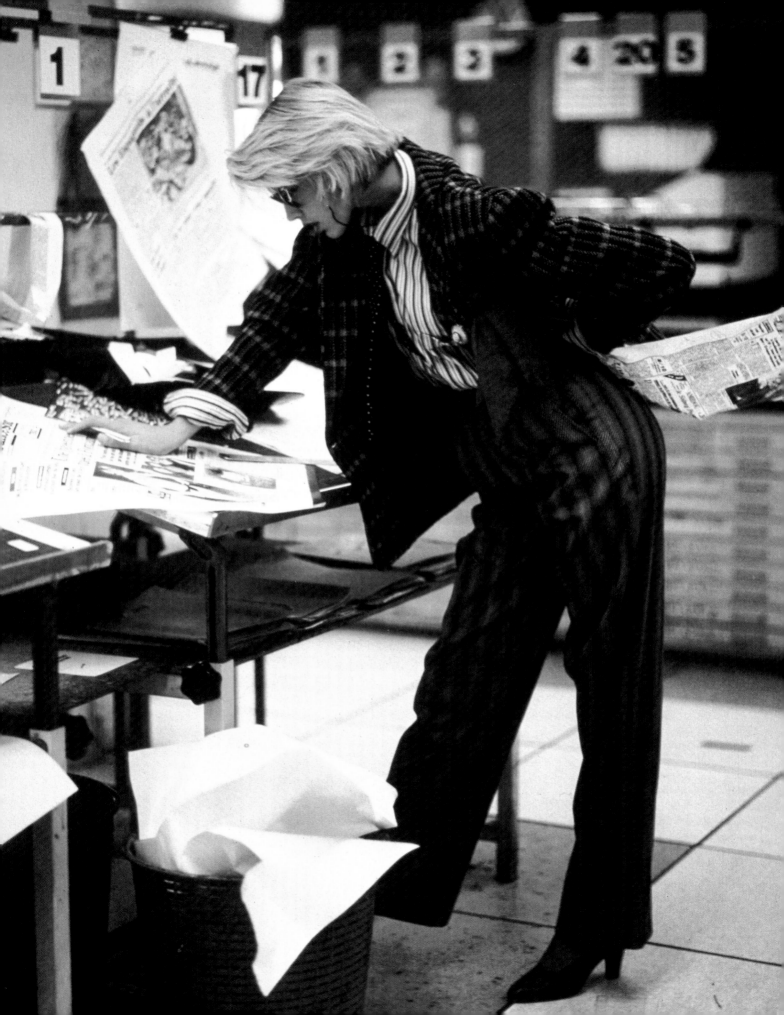

WORK TIME

Work time should be a time for joy, a time to explore the challenges of each day and stretch yourself to meet them. Unfortunately, for many of us work becomes routine, with too few exciting challenges and too many tedious tasks – not to mention the stress induced by workplace politics and power struggles. To make work *good* for you, you need to be 'lucky' – which is to say that you need to be doing a job which gives you enough scope to make something of it and of yourself. But, strange as it may seem, much of this 'luck' depends, not on fate, but on your own expectations and on how much you value yourself (see p. 134).

To experience work as a pleasure rather than as a chore also means learning how to manage stress well, how to manipulate your work environment to your advantage – be it an office, a factory, a hospital, a shop or a studio – and how to eliminate as many of the environmental hazards which contribute to poor health and low energy levels as possible. You must also make the best possible use of breaks and lunch hours, and ensure that work takes its proper place in balance with the other sides of your life.

One of the most taxing aspects of work can be the simple question of getting there. Commuting needn't be stressful, provided you develop ways of using the time and distance to do other things, such as exercise or meditation.

Many of us, particularly ambitious or successful women, find that work becomes the be-all and end-all of life – something which, because it is done well, is used as a refuge from facing our own inner being and confronting the challenges of personal growth. The reasoning goes something like this: 'If I can just keep working hard enough and long enough, then everything will be just fine.' Well, it won't. Sooner or later the other aspects of your life, and perhaps even your work, will catch up with you and need to be wrestled with. None of us is a static being. Each of us is involved in a continuous, dynamic process of development – physically, intellectually, emotionally and spiritually.

Regard work as a part of that development and keep it in its proper place. Do not allow it to become a protection against the uncertainties of personal change, as some workaholics do. Wherever you work and whatever kind of work you do, the job-related guidelines discussed in this chapter will help you get the most from your life. They can help you take pride in your work and in yourself. Use them together with some of the other techniques in this book and join the lucky ones who get up each morning looking forward to the work day, even if until now you've never felt this way.

ENVIRONMENTAL CHALLENGE

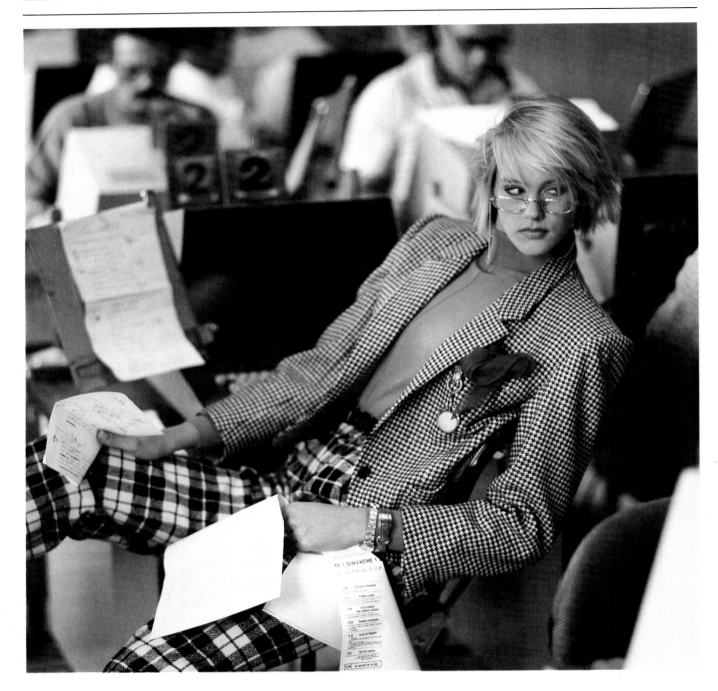

Finding the time for healthy good looks can be a real challenge for anyone with a nine-to-five job. At the end of a gruelling day at work, the last thing you are going to want to do is jump into a tracksuit and pound the pavements for half an hour. The *Time Alive* trick is to use your working day productively, incorporating energy-building routines along the way, so that you end up with energy to spare. Then all you need to do is freshen up and have fun!

THE HOSTILE OFFICE ENVIRONMENT
The first step towards maximizing your work time is to become aware just how your work environment affects your mood and health. Even in offices, many factors – lack of fresh air, copier chemicals, dust from carbonless copy paper, fluorescent lighting and VDU (visual display unit) radiation – can take their toll on your health, vitality and good looks. One or more of these may be responsible for that headache, your chronic tiredness or those

other mysterious symptoms – from irritated eyes to skin rashes – which develop at work. Clinical ecologists (doctors concerned with the effect of environment on human health) increasingly refer to such phenomena as the 'indoor climate syndrome'. Unfortunately, in most work-place environments, it can be hard to pin-point just what is responsible for a particular reaction. The best way of coping is to protect yourself as much as possible on a broad front.

● **Light up your life** Fluorescent lighting emits a flicker which can disturb the nervous system of some people, causing tension and headaches. Most artificial lighting is very different from natural light, which provides the full spectrum of light needed by your body to maintain a high level of health and well-being. Studies show that where work-place fluorescent lighting has been changed to special full-spectrum lighting people suffer less from chronic ailments, rates of absenteeism improve and morale is heightened. You may not be able to alter the lighting in the building where you work, but you can purchase a full-spectrum table light for your desk and perhaps even shut off the overhead light in your area. If the problem is serious, clip every newspaper or magazine story you see which reports new findings about the effects of light on health, and see that they make it on to your boss's desk.

● **Clear the air** You can also improve the quality of the air you breathe by placing a small ionizer on your desk. An ionizer sends negatively charged particles of air into the atmosphere, which can have a beneficial effect on how you feel and function, much as if you were standing by a waterfall or by the sea, where the air is also charged by negative ions. The air in most urban environments, particularly in buildings made from cement, either is largely depleted of all ions or contains a high percentage of positively charged ions – both of which seem to have a negative effect on health. Many migraine headaches, respiratory problems and colds can be avoided by breathing ionized air, which also improves concentration and helps keep you even-tempered.

Cigarettes contribute enormously to atmospheric pollution, for non-smokers as well as for smokers. Keep away from people who smoke. Tell the people you live and work with that you are bothered by cigarette smoke and ask them please not to smoke. (Since everybody

seems to respect 'doctor's orders', tell smokers that you are *allergic* to smoke to make it easier for them to comply with your wishes.) If you must be in a room with someone who is smoking, make sure it is well ventilated. The anti-oxidant nutrients (see pp. 108–9) can help protect you from much of the damage that can be caused by cigarette smoke.

● **Radiation is no joke** Word processors and computers are wonderful work-savers. But they also emit continuous, low-level electromagnetic radiation which can be detrimental to health. As a result, some countries now regulate the amount of time an operator is allowed to work without a break at a VDU or prevent pregnant women from using them at all.

If you work with a computer or word processor, get up and walk around for a few minutes after each hour. Make sure you have plenty of the anti-oxidant nutrients to help protect your body from free radical damage and the excessive oxidation that can result from even low levels of radiation.

Be aware that there are hazards in the work-place, otherwise you might think there's something wrong with you because you feel depressed every time you walk into the office. If you are in a job with serious health risks and it is not possible to improve conditions, then it is worth putting your health first and finding a new job.

PROTECT YOURSELF

○ When typing or working at a VDU, avoid backache by sitting with your back straight and your feet firmly planted on the floor.

○ Keep photocopying machines and printers in separate rooms from the ones you work in.

○ Make sure that VDU screens are placed at a right angle to any light source, such as a lamp or window, to minimize reflected glare, which causes fatigue and headaches. If necessary, fit an anti-glare screen over the VDU screen.

○ Store carbonless copy paper in a closed cupboard to avoid breathing in its fumes.

○ Try not to create dust – say, by tearing up paper – and keep your work-place as clean as possible.

○ See that your office is well ventilated and no hotter than 67–68°F (20°C).

THE RUSH CRUSH

For many people the most stressful and draining part of the day is travelling to and from work during the rush hour. Just the thought of all those impatient pushing bodies trying to get ahead is enough to exhaust anyone. If you're lucky enough to work special hours and can avoid the rush – so much the better. If not, then here are some tips to help you make the most of your travel time. The first thing to realize is that, whether you're on a bus or train or in a car, no amount of fretting and looking at your watch is going to help you get where you're going any quicker. So you might as well relax.

COMMUTING BY CAR

If you drive to work, you are at least assured of a seat and a few square feet of space. It is an ideal time to listen to music, or you might like to sing along to songs by your favourite vocalist. Singing is ideal for de-stressing: it lifts your spirits and helps you relax physically by increasing the depth of your breathing. Don't mind any strange looks from other motorists – more often than not they will laugh to see you talking to yourself, and smiles among the rush hour scowls are another welcome relief.

Driving in traffic is a time to pace yourself and keep calm inside. The aggression and frustration of the other drivers trapped in traffic can be contagious. Some motorists feel it their responsibility to tell you which lane you should be in or to let you know when you've made a mistake, and it is tempting to over-react if someone honks at you. But don't be rattled. Learn to stay calm and let over-anxious motorists take care of their own driving.

When the traffic light turns red just as you approach it, don't get frustrated and try to race through. Instead, stop, relax and take a few seconds simply to breathe. Notice your posture. If you are anxiously gripping the steering wheel or craning your neck forward, sit back in your seat and wait for the light to change. Remember – glaring at it won't make it change any faster. Instead, practise the Breath of Life exercise and your de-stressing command (see p. 72).

ON THE BUS OR TRAIN

If you can sit down, a bus or train ride can be quite enjoyable. A journey of 20 minutes or more gives you time for a meditation or relaxation exercise. Make yourself comfortable, if possible in a seat where you will not have to move. If you like, listen to peaceful music on a portable radio or cassette tape player with head-phones. Don't worry about people watching – a 'sleeping' person is a decidedly uninteresting sight. If you're on your way to work, try a breathing meditation based on the Breath of Life exercise to give you energy and wake you up. Imagine that you breathe in energy or light and breathe away fatigue and tension. If you're on your way home, try the Bubble Meditation, a simple visualization exercise to clear your mind of all the day's worries and leave work far behind.

● **The Bubble Meditation** Close your eyes and give a deep sigh. Become aware of any tensions in your forehead, neck, shoulders and the rest of your body and let them go. Let your breathing become calm and steady. Imagine your mind as a pool of carbonated water and any thought that comes into it as a bubble which floats out of your consciousness, fading in the distance. The bubbles may be pieces of office gossip, worries about what you're going to eat for dinner or a reminder that you have to send someone a birthday card. Label each one and watch it float up and out of your mind. Gradually, the bubbles will come more slowly, until you are left with a still, clear mind. Enjoy this feeling of peace and clear-headedness and you can open your eyes refreshed.

● **If you don't get a seat** Even if you aren't lucky enough to get a seat on the train or bus, you can still take advantage of the journey time. The worst thing about standing on a bus or train is being jostled or pushed by the crowd. Protect yourself and conserve your energy with this simple mind-over-matter trick: as you walk to your stop, or while you're waiting there, imagine that you are enclosed in a protective layer of coloured light. Visualize this protective layer surrounding you and shielding you from your environment. When you get on the train or bus, reinforce the first layer with a second one. This may sound esoteric, but no matter how much you are jostled and pushed, you won't feel so exposed or get so exhausted. Try it. Another good exercise to do while standing at the stop or on the bus or train is 'rooting', which will plant your feet so firmly that they'll support you no matter how tired you feel.

● **Plant your feet firmly** Because of anxiety or restrictive shoes, most of us fail to establish good contact with

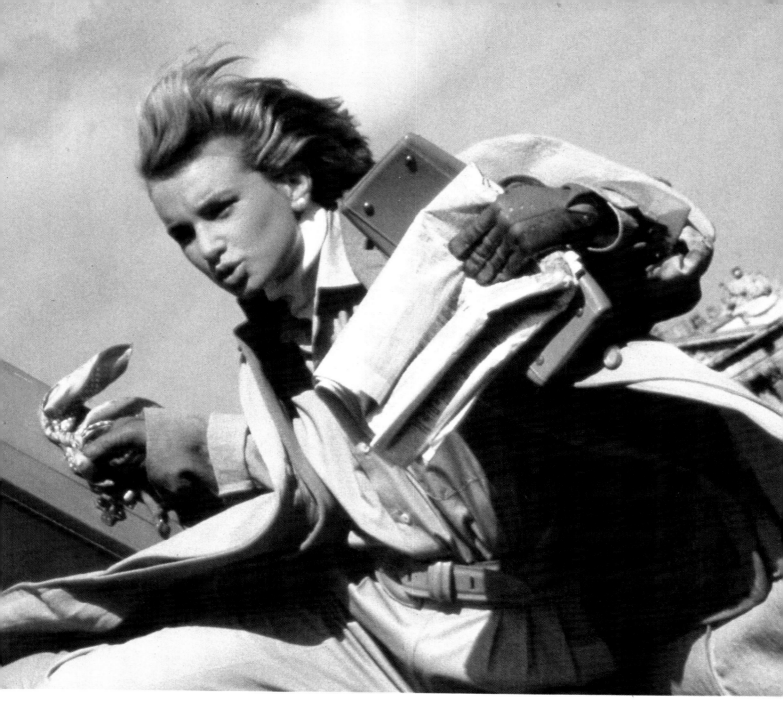

the ground. But good contact is vital to your posture, your breathing and even your thinking. Use this exercise to plant your feet firmly and they'll support you no matter how tired you feel. After a minute or two, your spine will align itself naturally, so you look and feel refreshed.

Stand comfortably with your feet shoulder-width apart. Imagine that you have roots growing down through the soles of your feet. Try to visualize strong thick roots which penetrate the ground and grow down to a depth as great as your own height, anchoring you firmly. At the same time imagine the top of your head lifting up towards the sky. As your spine lengthens you will feel greater space in your chest and back, your muscles will relax and your breathing will become full and easy. The more clearly you can visualize your roots,

the better this exercise will work. If you have difficulty in imagining this get a piece of paper and draw yourself with roots growing from the soles of your feet so that you will be able to see the image more clearly in your mind's eye.

ON FOOT

One easy way to incorporate exercise into your day is to bicycle to and from work, or to skip public transport and walk part of your journey in comfortable flat shoes. High heels only contribute to muscle tension and poor circulation – and thus to stress. If you carry a shoulder bag, the strap should cross your body, not just hang from one shoulder, to help guard against backache. Better still, carry a back-pack-type bag with straps over both shoulders which distribute the weight evenly.

THE BREAKS

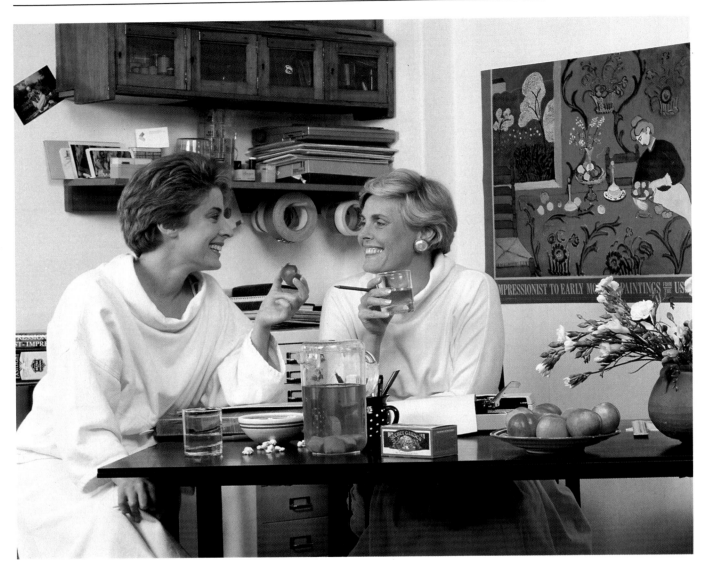

For most workers the breaks are few and far between. The day consists of seven hours of work with a one-hour break for lunch and at best an afternoon tea break or morning coffee break. With so little time to breathe, it's vital that you make your breaks work *for* you, not against you.

TEA OR COFFEE BREAKS

These may be official breaks or simply a chance to grab a quick cup of something between phone calls or other tasks. Average consumption of tea or coffee can range from a single cup in the morning to six or more cups a day. For most people, having another cup becomes an automatic response. The problem is that, after the initial caffeine pick-up, tea or coffee can let you down badly.

Few people know or want to know how much damage a few cups of tea or coffee a day can do. Both tea and coffee contain caffeine, a drug from the xanthine group of chemicals: about 90–120 mg of caffeine per cup of coffee and about 40–100 mg per cup of tea. Caffeine stimulates the central nervous system, pancreas and heart, as well as the cerebral cortex. This is why a cup of tea or coffee will give you a *temporary* boost in energy, but after its short-lived effects wear off, your blood-sugar level will drop lower than it was to begin with and you will feel exhausted. So you reach for a second cup and a vicious cycle begins.

An average tea or coffee consumption of a few cups a day has been linked with such complaints as heart disorders, high blood pressure, atherosclerosis, gastric ulcers and even mental illness. Caffeine can cause your heart to beat rapidly and irregularly, increase the level of free fatty acids in your blood, stimulate the excretion of excess acid in your stomach and raise your blood pressure. Recent studies have identified a phenomenon known as 'caffeinism', which links caffeine intake by habitual coffee-drinkers to mental illnesses – from quite simple depression and anxiety neurosis to overt psychosis. In an already stressful office environment, a cup of tea or coffee will only contribute to general fatigue and edginess in the long run. Look instead to natural, energy-boosting drinks to sustain you through the day.

THE CAFFEINE-FREE BREAK
Our favourite pick-up drink is a glass of vitamin C tonic. We once kept a three-day meeting peppy by continually topping up everyone's glasses with our tonic. No one touched the tea and coffee provided and we completely forgot to take tea and coffee breaks. To make the tonic simply add about ½ teaspoon (1–2 grams) of powdered vitamin C to a glass of plain or fizzy spring water and sweeten it with a little clear honey or raw sugar. Or stir the vitamin C into a glass of fruit juice, such as apple, grape or pineapple.

If you prefer a hot drink, make a delicious cup of hot, spiced apple juice by adding boiling water and a pinch of cinnamon to apple juice concentrate (the cinnamon is great for settling a stomach). Or try a barley/chicory coffee substitute. (Due to the way it's processed, 'decaffeinated' coffee is not a good alternative.)

Wonderful herbal tea combinations, ranging in flavour from almond to cranberry, are sold in convenient sachets. Just add boiling water and allow the herbal tea to steep for several minutes for full flavour. If you like, add a little clear honey as sweetener. Some herbs, such as lemon grass, are particularly helpful for pepping you up, while others, such as camomile, soothe your nerves. Have both types around.

If you're lucky enough to have a centrifuge juicer, squeeze fresh juice, such as carrot or apple, in the morning and keep it in a vacuum flask or Thermos with

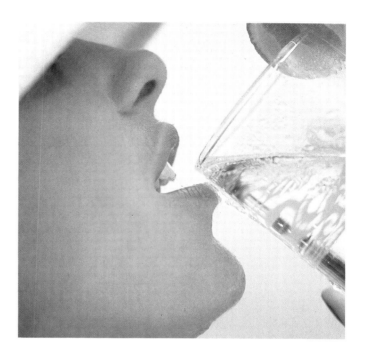

ice to drink throughout the day. Although they are a hassle to make, freshly squeezed juices make the most wonderful pick-up drinks. Or simply keep a bottle of plain or carbonated spring water to drink at work. Most offices can be very dehydrating and replenishing body fluids is an important health booster.

SNACK TIME
Even those of us who care about eating well can fall down on between-meal snacks. You're most inclined to eat something you may later regret when you're hungry. Rather than trying to avoid eating between meals, it's best to allow for those mid-morning or mid-afternoon cravings and keep a healthy snack on hand to stop you from gobbling a chocolate bar. We often keep a mixture of raisins or sultanas with sunflower and/or pumpkin seeds stashed in a small cottage cheese container in our handbags. Homemade popcorn is also a healthy, favourite snack. Always carry one or two crunchy apples to work, especially for the mid-morning snack. If we know our hectic schedule won't permit a decent lunch, we often just carry apples with us to eat during the day. They are quick, convenient and sustaining. Then we can have our main meal in the evening.

If you have an overwhelming craving for chocolate, try carob, the healthy alternative. You can buy dark brown, unrefined carob pods with their seeds inside (sometimes called St John's Bread) from good health food shops. Simply chew on the pods whenever you get the chocolate urge. If you constantly crave sweet things, it may be because your system is depleted of the B-complex vitamins, so try taking a teaspoon of unsulphured blackstrap molasses. It is rich in B-complex vitamins and will also satisfy your sweet craving.

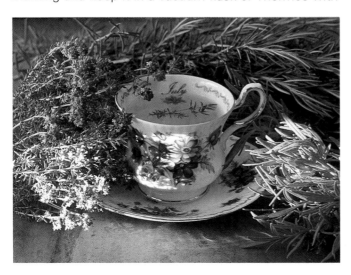

THE LUNCH BOOST

Make a conscious effort to shift down a gear for lunch, or you may find yourself eating your lunch to the rhythm of your typewriter and suffering from indigestion. Step out of the office for a welcome breather walking in a park or visiting an art gallery. Don't take your office work to lunch with you by worrying over a problem. Leave it behind and come back to it with a fresh mind later.

Take care about what you eat. On top of a hectic morning, the wrong lunch can make your afternoon a misery. Consider how you will feel in an hour or so before you grab a chocolate bar or some greasy fast food. Avoid the energy drainers listed below.

DIGEST AID

If a heavy work-day lunch has left you feeling bloated and fatigued, don't despair. Try this remedy: take a digestive enzyme supplement (available from most health food shops) with a high-potency vitamin B pill and a glass of vitamin C tonic (see p. 69) when you get back to work. A piece of fresh fruit, such as pineapple, or a cup of peppermint tea, can also be helpful.

HIGH-ENERGY LUNCHES

If you really want to triumph over the mid-afternoon slump, then look to a high-energy lunch. Because raw foods contain certain valuable enzymes, they are far less taxing on the digestive system than their cooked counterparts and you can use your energy for your work, rather than for digesting your lunch. Any fresh raw fruits and vegetables thus make a good basis for an ideal lunch. Depending on where your work-place is located, you may be able to find fresh salads at a nearby delicatessen or café.

Often the simplest lunches are the best. A couple of pieces of fresh fruit (remember to wash or wipe it clean) with a carton of plain goat's or sheep's milk yoghurt or cottage cheese make a delicious and sustaining lunch. Or try some fresh fruit and a granola muesli bar with unrefined sugar or honey. If you carry your lunch to work, crudités are ideal. Dips are a great way to give variety to a lunch of raw vegetable and fruit crudités. Cut up vegetables of all sorts, such as carrots, celery, sweet green peppers, cucumber, red cabbage or cauliflower, and pack them in an airtight box together with a small carton of homemade dip. Or you can mix a low-calorie dressing by putting one cup (225 g) of tofu (soya

bean curd), the juice of a lemon, one teaspoon (5 ml) each of honey and fresh grated ginger root, one pressed garlic clove and one tablespoon (15 ml) of red wine into a processor and blending well. Also bring some fresh fruit and, if you feel like you need something more substantial, a wholemeal roll or muffin, rye crackers or Scottish oatcakes.

DIPS FOR PACKED LUNCHES

Delicious raw dips are a great way to give variety to a lunch of raw vegetable and fruit crudités. All of the ones given here can be made up in just a few minutes with a blender or a food processor (without one it takes a little longer). Once made, most will keep for a few days in the refrigerator, so you can make a batch to last for three or four lunches. Many of the recipes call for vegetable bouillon powder, which can be found in most health food stores. The measurements are meant to be rough guidelines. Use your imagination and experiment. If you don't have a particular ingredient, improvise!

ENERGY DRAINERS

○ **Fried lunch**
Greasy fried food – fish and chips, hamburgers, bacon and eggs – is most likely of all to send you to sleep because meals heavy in fat sludge your blood and slow down your mental processes.

○ **Pizza and pasta**
The combination of carbohydrate (pasta and pizza base) with protein (meat or cheese) makes these foods very difficult to digest. In addition, they are usually made with white flour, which robs your body of the B-complex vitamins you need to cope with stress and fatigue.

○ **Liquid lunch**
One danger of lunching in a wine bar, pub or restaurant (whatever other energy-draining consequences it might have) is that you will have a few glasses of wine or beer as well. Alcohol, like refined sugar, will give you a temporary buzz and then leave you with low blood-sugar and a resulting mid-afternoon slump.

○ **Sandwiches**
Often eaten in haste, sandwiches are not a particularly good choice, unless they are made from wholemeal bread and are not heavily plastered with butter or mayonnaise.

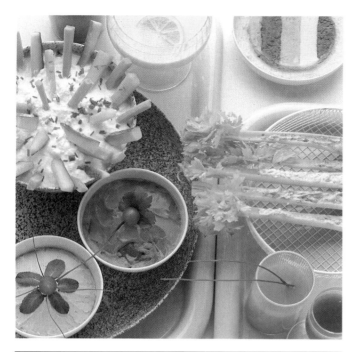

Avocado/Orange Dip

This is our number one favourite dip. When avocados are in season and cheap, it's a real treat!

1 ripe avocado
4 fl oz (½ cup/120 ml) fresh orange juice
2 tsp (10 ml) vegetable bouillon powder
1 tsp (5 ml) mild curry powder
fresh herbs, such as parsley and chives
1 small clove garlic (optional)

Halve the avocado, remove the stone and scoop out the flesh. Blend all the ingredients together in a food processor or mash by hand until smooth, adding enough orange juice to achieve the desired consistency. Store in an airtight container in the refrigerator until needed. The fresh orange juice helps to preserve this dip, but it should be eaten within two days.

Carrot/Nutmeg Dip

1–2 carrots, roughly chopped
8 oz (1 cup/225 g) cottage cheese
a handful of walnuts or sunflower seeds
½ tsp (2.5 ml) nutmeg
a handful of fresh parsley
a pinch of vegetable bouillon powder
a little water, to thin

Blend the carrots well in the processor along with the cottage cheese and nuts or seeds. Add the herbs and seasonings and a little water to thin.

Greek Cucumber Dip

This dip is best when you make it with sheep's yoghurt.

a handful of sunflower seeds
½ large cucumber
8 fl oz (1 cup/225 ml) thick yoghurt
1 tsp (5 ml) French mustard
1 tsp (5 ml) honey
½ tsp (2.5 ml) crushed dried dill
½ tsp (2.5 ml) crushed dried coriander seed
a few leaves of fresh mint or 1 tsp (5 ml) dried
vegetable bouillon powder, to taste

Grind the sunflower seeds finely in the food processor. Peel the cucumber and chop roughly. Put in the processor with the other ingredients and mix well.

Sprouted Humous Dip

You can, of course, make humous in the traditional way, with cooked chickpeas, but we prefer the flavour of sprouted chickpeas. It only takes three days to grow your own chickpea sprouts: soak chickpeas overnight in a bowl of water, then rinse and drain in a jar or seed tray. Leave them in a warm place and rinse and drain them once or twice a day. At the end of three days or when they are about 1 in (2 cm) long, you should have delicious sprouts to eat in salads, wok-fry with vegetables or use in this delicious dip. Tahini (finely ground sesame seed paste) is available from delicatessens.

8 fl oz (1 cup/225 ml) chickpea sprouts
2 Tbsp (30 ml) olive oil
juice of one lemon
2 Tbsp (30 ml) tahini
1 clove garlic
1–2 tsp (5–10 ml) vegetable bouillon powder
a little water, to thin
½ tsp (2.5 ml) paprika

Blend the sprouts very finely in the food processor. Add the oil, lemon juice, tahini, garlic and bouillon powder, and blend, with water if needed. Spoon into an airtight storage container and top with paprika.

STRESS RELEASE

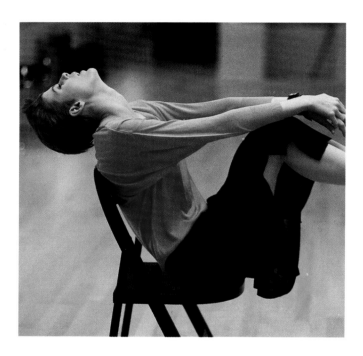

The first step in dealing with stress is recognizing its signs in your body. We all have specific areas where we hold onto tension. Usually you are not aware of these tensions because your body adapts to them and considers them the norm. You only discover a tension when it becomes so severe that it actually causes you pain. If you can locate the areas in your body which tend to be tight, you can unload not only the physical tension but also the emotional and mental stress you are carrying around. Once you're free of those burdens, you will cope much more easily with demands made on you.

YOUR TENSION AREAS

As you are reading this, become aware of your body. Notice your face, for instance. Are your lips tightly closed? Are you clenching your jaw? Are you scowling? At first it is often difficult to locate the areas of your body where you hold onto tension. In your free time at home, try the following simple technique for discovering the tense spots.

Lie down on your back on the floor with a pillow supporting your head and bend your knees comfortably, keeping the soles of your feet on the floor. Become aware of your breathing and focus your concentration

on each part of your body, beginning with your head and working down to your feet. A tight spot will often feel 'dull' or seem 'dark' because tense muscles reduce sensitivity in that area. For the moment don't do anything about the tension, just observe it.

Once you have discovered your particular areas of tension, say, for example, your neck and shoulders, focus on one area and imagine your worries, like paying the phone bill or finishing off a piece of work, as burdens hanging onto your shoulders. Then imagine a warmth and softness spreading through your shoulders which melts the burdens away as you breathe. On each out-breath, you release a little more. As you do this, you may find that tension in another part of your body disappears as well. That will help you discover another of your typical holding areas.

After you have identified your holding areas, you can use this exercise throughout the day, whether you're sitting or in motion, to let go of tension. You can also prevent yourself from taking on tensions by anticipating your physical reaction to a stressor. For example, if someone shouts at you, take a moment to think, breathe out and release your typical holding areas. Refuse to allow stress to become a personal burden. Let the other person's aggression flow off you like water off a duck's back.

YOUR DE-STRESSING COMMAND

Choose one or two personal de-stressing commands. Every word or phrase has a slightly different connotation for each person, so it is important that your command works for you. An example might be, 'My shoulders are heavy and my head is calm and clear.' Whichever words bring about the relaxation response for you are best. Some helpful images are: warm, soft, heavy, free, easy, calm, regular, melt, float. Once you have chosen a de-stressor command use it regularly. The more you practise letting go, the easier it will become.

THE BREATH OF LIFE

How you feel is almost always reflected in the way you breathe. When you experience emotional extremes, such as laughing or crying, your breathing also becomes extreme. Likewise, by changing your breathing pattern, you can affect the way you feel. In this way, breathing can be an important tool for de-stressing. Repeat the following simple breathing technique throughout the day to help you let go of tensions and get an energy pick-up.

Start by breathing in and out fully with a sigh. Wait for the in-breath to come by itself. As the air comes in, imagine that the breath is energy reviving you. Let it fill out your abdomen first, and then your chest. Don't raise your shoulders. Then, as you breathe out again, imagine you are exhaling all the tension and stress in your body and let your muscles relax. Pause, breathe in once more and then continue with whatever you were doing. Use the Breath of Life exercise whenever you experience a stress trigger, say, when you hear the telephone ring or catch yourself looking at your watch if you're late. Stick a brightly coloured tab on your watch strap and on your telephone to remind you to breathe, every time you see them.

THE TERRIBLE TELEPHONE

For most workers, a ringing telephone is one of the worst stressors. One phone call can upset your plans for the entire day. Most of us have unconsciously built up a negative attitude to the telephone, so that we are unnecessarily tense whenever we pick up the receiver. To combat this unwelcome tension, develop good telephone habits:

- When the phone rings don't answer it on the first ring. Instead, pause, breathe out and then pick it up. This will help you remember your own pacing and even give the person on the other end a chance to breathe out too.
- Rest the elbow of the hand holding the phone on your desk so that your arm is relaxed.
- Let your other arm relax by your side unless you need it for writing.
- When you are making a call be sure you are comfortable in your chair and relaxed. Breathe out before you dial.
- While you are waiting for the other person to answer, let go of any tensions in your throat, neck and shoulders. When your throat is relaxed, your voice sounds clear and assured. If you breathe from your diaphragm (not high in your chest), you shouldn't get a frog in your throat.

PEN PUSH-UPS

Although the work-place is not suitable for an enthusiastic aerobic work-out, there are some exercises which you can do sitting at your desk to revive you when you experience an energy slump. Select one or two to do at a time.

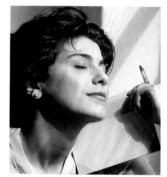

Neck Release
Let your head drop forwards so that your chin rests on your chest. Clasp your hands behind your head and gently let the weight of your arms pulling down lengthen out the spaces between the vertebrae in your neck. Then drop your head backwards and let your mouth drop open. Open and close your mouth like a fish and feel the stretch in your throat, which is great for toning up the neck and getting rid of a double chin. Bring your head back to centre and drop it to the left so that your ear dips towards your shoulder. Wrap the left arm over your head and gently help ease it down. Then ease your head over to the right side using the right arm. Circle your head slowly clockwise twice and then anti-clockwise twice. Finish by giving yourself a quick neck rub. Place your fingertips on either side of your neck vertebrae and rub up and down with small circular movements.

Shoulder Shrug
Lift your arms above your head, clasp your fingers and squeeze your shoulders up to your ears. Hold them there for a count of 5, then relax. Now push your shoulders as far back as possible, squeezing your shoulder-blades together for a count of 5, then relax. Rotate one shoulder backwards as if you are

unscrewing the upper arm away from the body, creating a space between your arm and the side of your body. Repeat with the other shoulder. Now take a breath in and imagine your torso widening and your upper arms moving even further away from each other. Maintain this distance as you breathe out. Repeat twice more.

Scalp Tap
For a quick energy boost, simply use your fingertips to tap lightly over the entire area of your skull. Some areas are sensitive, so tap lightly. Other areas, like the base of the skull, can benefit from a firmer tap. After tapping your skull, massage along the jaw bone, from below the ears to the chin. You may prefer to massage with small circular movements rather than tapping. Your whole head and face should feel alive and refreshed.

Eye Refresher
Lean your elbows on your desk and cup your hands over your closed eyes. Hold for about a minute, then gently release your hands and open your eyes. Blink several times. Repeat this exercise whenever your eyes are sore or tired. Remember to lubricate your eyes by blinking often if you are reading or working at a VDU.

DAZZLING URBANITE

You are not at your freshest at the end of a long, hard day. Yet you need only a few minutes to spare and a freshen-up kit to transform yourself from a drab office worker to a sparkling charmer – without even needing to touch base at home! After all, if Superwoman can do it, then so can you!

CLOTHING

● **Accessorize for glamour** Lugging a second wardrobe to work is not much fun, so it is usually best to wear the same clothes for your evening out that you wear by day. But it is easy to carry one or two accessories, such as a scarf or a belt, and fresh stockings or underwear. Jewellery is another easy way to dress up an outfit, especially bold earrings.

● **No sweat** Whether you call it glowing, perspiring or just plain old sweating, it is something which everyone does to a greater or lesser extent. Sweating, like breathing, is an important body process, helping eliminate wastes and cooling the body down when it gets too warm.

Try to wear clothes made from natural fibres, such as cotton, wool, linen and silk, which will allow your skin to breathe. About $\frac{1}{60}$th of the body's respiration – the process of absorbing oxygen and getting rid of poisonous gases – occurs through the skin. The role of skin in respiration is so important that covering the skin completely with a non-porous material such as spray paint leads to death within just a few hours. If you wear clothes made from synthetic materials you decrease the possibility of breathing through the entire surface of the skin and you may actually find you don't feel well as a result of this 'insulation'.

Never attempt to stop your body from sweating. Anti-perspirants are definitely a *no*. They prevent wastes from leaving the body, forcing them to seek another way out – often through the skin as pimples or spots. Many anti-perspirants contain aluminium salts which can cause heavy metal toxicity if they enter the body. Use a deodorant instead of an anti-perspirant – there is a difference. A deodorant permits perspiration, but neutralizes any unpleasant odour. The sweat of a truly healthy person will not smell bad at all, but even the healthiest person may want to use a deodorant in a polluted environment.

Foot odour, too, can be a problem. Sprinkle a little talcum powder into your shoes or use insoles containing charcoal to absorb any odour. If you have very bad foot odour, it may be due to a zinc deficiency. If you also have white marks on your nails or a cracked tongue, it is worth taking 25–50 mg of zinc per day for a few months.

TO THE MIRROR

Find yourself a spot in the women's room in front of a mirror. Don't feel rushed. Take a moment to breathe and loosen up your neck and shoulders.

● **Hair** Take a look at your hair. Give it a good brush or comb. If you are not pleased with it, change it. If you usually wear your long hair up, wear it down; if you wear it down during the day, try clipping it up with a twist at the back or pulling it back with a side comb on one or both sides. A ribbon or thin scarf tied around your head in a large bow can look fun. For short hair, it may be helpful to use a hair curler – the compact types that run on butane gas are excellent and very convenient to carry in a bag. Some hairstyles benefit from a freshen-up with a little hair gel rubbed between the palms and then smoothed over the hair to help fix it. If you are really unhappy with your hair or didn't have time to wash it in the morning, wrap it up, turban-like, with a scarf and tuck the ends in for a clean, dramatic look.

● **Teeth** We carry a toothbrush, toothpaste and some dental floss to help freshen up. A travel toothbrush which fits into a little plastic compact will stay clean and dry in your purse. Somehow when your mouth is clean you feel renewed.

● **Freshen up your face** Clean off any make-up smudges and wipe your lips clean with a cotton bud or a tissue. Rather than removing and reapplying your make-up (if you wear it), use a water spritzer to freshen it up and restore some moisture to your skin. Either buy a small atomizer of spring water especially for this, or carry the top part of a plant mister and use it with a cup of water. Clip your hair back from your face if necessary and spray your whole face and neck lightly with a mist of water to feel fresh again. A little water sprayed on permed, wavy or coarse hair can help pick up the curls. Allow your face to dry. If your eyes are tired, use some eye drops. Then touch up your make-up. A litte translucent face powder brushed over your cheeks and eye sockets will make a good base for your blusher. Take a

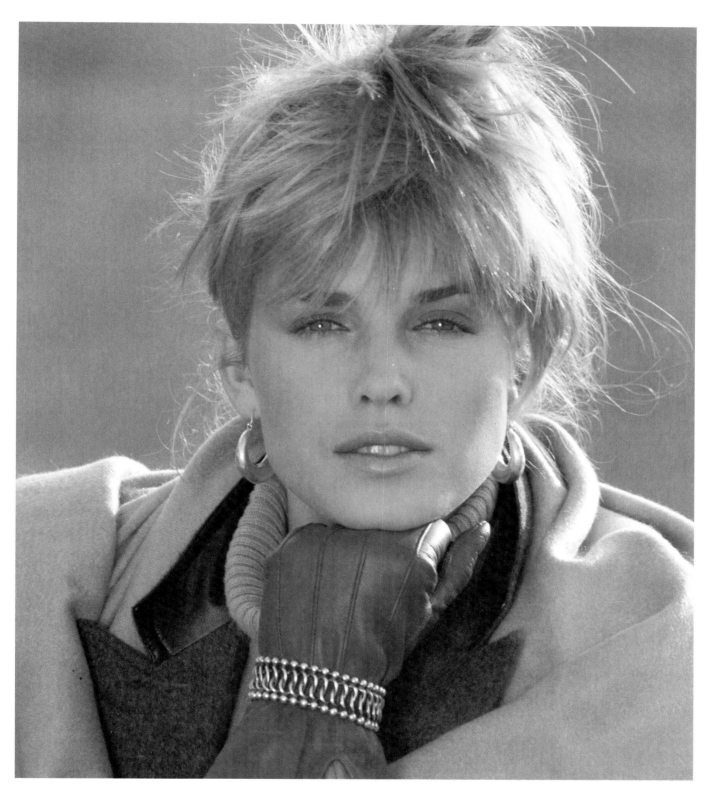

flattering blusher – dusty pink or apricot – and fluff it lightly on to your cheeks, chin and eye sockets. Touch up your eyes with a little mascara and eye-liner. Renew your lipstick by applying one layer, blotting it and then applying a second. A fresh shade of lipstick will help you register that work time is over.

For a glamorous evening look, brush shimmery gold or silver highlighter above your cheek bones and onto your brow bones below the eyebrows. Use a little in the inner corners of the eye to make the eyes sparkle. Accentuate the bow of your lips by putting a touch at the top of the lower lip and blending it in.

BEWARE SUPERWOMAN

Are you one of those miracle-working superwomen who hold down a demanding job from nine to five (or six, or seven) and then come home to look after home and family, care for relatives and friends? Do you shop, run errands and cook for partner or children and still expect yourself to emerge from it all as a stunning glamour girl? This is what we call playing the super-woman role – a role which is becoming commonplace with creative and ambitious women. It is a dangerous game to play. Push yourself beyond your limits too often, and you can begin to suffer physical symptoms such as headaches, colds or flu; back, neck and shoulder ache; or chronic fatigue and PMS (pre-menstrual syndrome).

Superwomen are no strangers to emotional troubles, especially feelings of inadequacy, depression and irritability. They are more inclined than most to develop a dependence on alcohol or drugs. Those who push themselves too hard eventually find that they are not doing their best, either in their work or for the people closest to them. Many an intimate relationship has failed as a result of the superwoman syndrome. Don't let it happen to you.

Whenever you suspect that the superwoman syndrome is creeping up on you, take a good look at the points listed below and make a few changes in your life.

REACH FOR THE TOP – NEVER STRUGGLE IN VAIN

Take a close look at your values. What really matters to you? Despite what women's magazines sometimes tell us, you *can't* have everything. Make choices and rejoice in the freedom that such choice-making will bring you. Otherwise you could end up no more than a worn-out work-horse fit only for the glue factory.

STOP DOING EVERYTHING YOURSELF

Start delegating chores, both at work and at home. Even the most adamant perfectionist must sooner or later enlist help. Whenever you can, get someone else to do what needs to be done.

DON'T SAY YES TO EVERYTHING

When something is asked of you, give yourself time to consider the request before you immediately agree. Is it something that you can handle with relative ease? What are you going to have to lay aside to do it? What is it going to cost you in terms of time? All these things need to be considered before you agree to any request, either at work or at home.

FORGET THE HERO IMAGE

Like many women you may assume that you are supposed to be able to do everything. You're not. You are only human. And you'd be surprised how much pleasure it can bring to other people when they feel they can do something for you for a change. Express your needs and many of them are likely to be satisfied. Lock them away behind the perfectly together super-woman and you go it alone.

GUARD YOUR TIME JEALOUSLY

Limit the time you spend on non-essential tasks and activities, such as seeing people you don't really like just because you feel it is expected of you. Cut back on chores you feel you have to do. Do you really *have* to? Couldn't somebody else do them for you? Or might they not remain undone for the sake of your peace of mind?

SORT YOUR PRIORITIES

Take a look at what is absolutely essential to your life and what is marginal. If you can, write your priorities down on a piece of paper. Then make sure the time and effort you spend is in line with your priorities. Take an active role in deciding how you will spend your time and live your life. Don't just let it happen.

CREATE A ROUTINE

From day to day you need to make sure you have enough time to relax, take care of yourself and spend time with the people you love. No partnership will flourish without time together. Relaxation, recreation and having fun are just as important as hard work, responsibility and success. Make sure you get the balance right.

HIRE WHEN YOU CAN

Consider forgoing that new dress or pair of shoes and spend the money instead on help around the house or on help with your family if you have one. This will free you for doing other things (preferably *not* more work). After all, you earn money to improve the quality of your life. Without time to enjoy it, there *is* no quality.

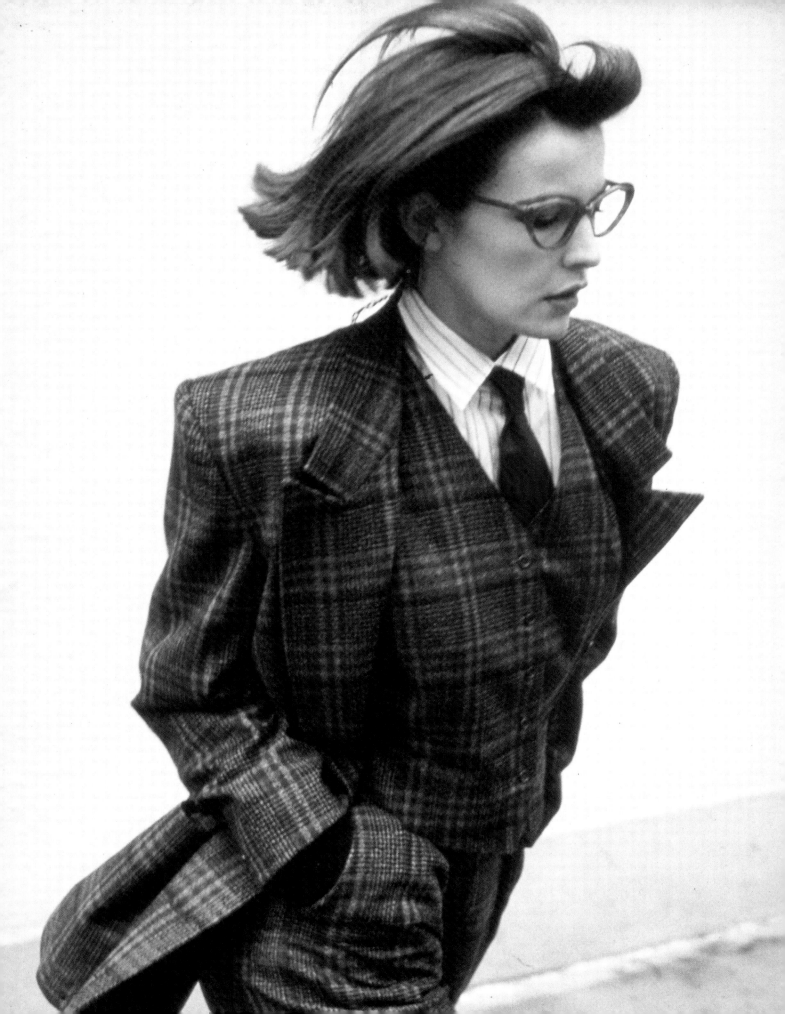

HAZARDOUS HABITS

Drugs, cigarettes and alcohol are forces to be reckoned with. Whatever their advantages may be in terms of assisting relaxation or altering consciousness, these are easily overshadowed by their disadvantages. Drugs are absolutely beyond the pale. Alcohol and cigarettes poison the body, muddle the mind and encourage premature aging and degeneration. What you may not know is that women appear to be more affected than men by all three – both positively and negatively.

FORGET THE CIGARETTES

Everybody knows that cigarette smoke contains many cancer-causing substances, such as nitrosamines, nitrogen dioxide, hydrogen cyanide, arsenic and formaldehyde, as well as tar, nicotine, carbon dioxide and ammonia. Cigarette smoking is also a major contributor to heart disease, emphysema, gastric ulcers and low birth-weight babies. Cigarette smoke interferes with good circulation and undermines your vitality. It suppresses your immune system and is particularly damaging to your skin, causing it to sag and age.

Even if you are not a cigarette smoker yourself, just being in an environment where cigarette smoke is present can cause you trouble.

● **Save your skin** Studies show that smokers have skin which is much more wrinkled than non-smokers'. This is because cigarettes deplete your body of vitamin C, zinc and the bioflavonoids, all of which are essential to formation of new collagen, the structural protein which gives your skin its form and youthful firmness. If you do smoke, you should take extra supplements to counteract this: about 10,000 IUs (international units) of vitamin A (best taken in the form of beta-carotene), at least 3 grams of vitamin C, at least 100 mg of the bioflavonoids and at least 25 mg of zinc.

● **Kicking the habit** Of course, it is far better to quit smoking altogether. Try carrying a bag of uncooked sunflower seeds in your pocket or handbag and reach for them whenever you feel the urge to smoke. Uncooked sunflower seeds are rich in most of the B-complex vitamins, vitamin E and essential fatty acids and contain ingredients which mimic some of nicotine's effects. Like nicotine, sunflower seeds have mildly soothing, sedative effects on the nervous system. Both substances also trigger the release of glycogen from the liver, producing a temporary increase in brain ac-

tivity, and both stimulate adrenal functions, thus raising the level of adrenal hormones in the body. But the differences between them are every bit as important as their similarities. Sunflower seeds, unlike cigarettes, are good for you. They can help break the negative addictive cigarette pattern without creating a new one.

THE DANGERS OF DRINK

A woman's capacity for drinking alcohol without becoming inebriated is about 30 per cent lower than a man's. Little alcohol tends to enter fat cells (thanks to their limited blood supply), so because a woman has more fat on her body, her lean tissues and organs (such as the liver and the brain) become flooded with alcohol sooner than a man's. Women are particularly vulnerable to the effects of alcohol near their menstrual period. At that time of the month you will probably do best to steer clear of alcohol altogether.

Work and alcohol can seem inextricably linked. There's the drink *before* lunch, then the wine *with* lunch, then the drink *after* work and drinks in the evening at home or out on the town with friends. For many women, this adds up to too much alcohol, and too much alcohol is dangerous. A study by American researchers which focussed on alcohol consumption equivalent to a business executive's average intake showed that heavy social drinking can *seriously* damage your liver, even though you may feel fine, act normally under the influence of alcohol and not be an alcoholic. Even subjects on a high-protein diet supplemented with vitamins experienced increases of 5–13 times in the level of fat in their livers after only eight days. Since then, a number of other studies have turned up similar results. That's the bad news.

The good news is this: researchers have also found that liver cell damage and the increase in fat levels in the liver are *reversible* if the drinker abstains from alcohol for long enough. But they warn that the long-term damage to the liver which results from the daily consumption of alcohol over the years can be *irreversible*. Persistent drinking can also, they say, lead to specific liver diseases, such as cirrhosis, to other toxic conditions and to premature aging.

● **Look after your liver** After your skin, your liver is your body's largest organ, and in many ways it is also the most important. You could live without a stomach, if necessary, but never without a liver. It is your body's chemical purifier, performing over 500 known functions. Many of these are concerned with detoxifying your body, cleansing it of all the drugs, pollutants and poisons you take in every day, including alcohol.

If your liver is overworked or 'worn out' by excess alcohol or drug consumption, eventually and *unavoidably* your whole body suffers. It was formerly thought that excess alcohol was no more damaging to the liver than too much sugar or too many rich foods – that the real damage to the liver came from malnutrition. These theories have been disproved. Both the *quantity* of alcohol you drink and the *duration* of serious drinking are important factors in determining liver damage.

● **The effect on the brain** Despite the immediate lift you feel when you take your first drink, alcohol is actually a *depressant*. It is rapidly absorbed through the digestive system and begins to act on the front part of your brain almost as soon as it hits your bloodstream, deadening and interfering with the specific centres which govern your self-control, judgement and inhibitions. This is the source of your transient feelings of well-being. Alcohol also stimulates stomach secretions, affects the central nervous system, affects circulation in the skin, causes diuresis and interferes with the co-ordination of your muscles, nerves and vision. It does have a tranquillizing effect and, because it tends to increase your desire for food, is useful in moderation for people who tend to suffer from poor appetite.

● **Practise moderation** So what's the answer to the alcohol dilemma? Do you become an anti-social tee-totaller, eschewing even the smallest drop? Or do you live in blind ignorance, drinking whatever you are offered because it's so hard to say 'no', even though you will wake the next morning feeling less than good and unable to function at your peak? These are questions each woman has to answer for herself. We take a middle line. Often we drink nothing. This is particularly easy in circles where it is fashionable to opt for mineral water with a twist of lemon or lime. Other times we enjoy drinking up to two or three glasses of wine with our meal. Occasionally, we drink a glass of naturally brewed, old-fashioned stout, which is rich in B-complex vitamins. But only rarely do we drink spirits – usually only at our annual family cocktail party, when we splash out and have two or even three exotic cocktails.

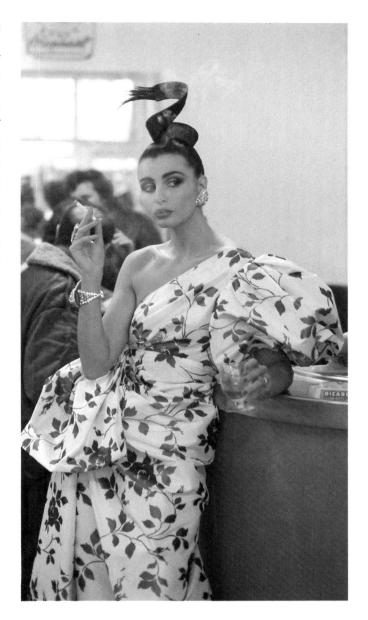

We almost never drink too much because both of us have experienced that feeling and neither of us likes it. We value our energy, our health and our good looks too much to jeopardize them for the sake of a social convention. If current practices and social conventions don't fit your needs, chances are there are others who feel the same way. So maybe it's time to change them.

DRINK YOUR HEALTH

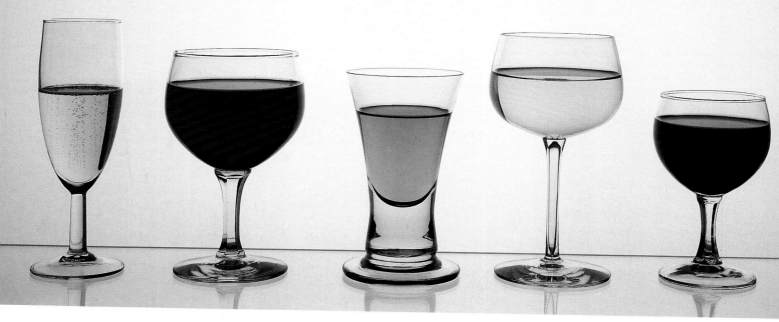

But don't get the idea that *all* alcoholic beverages are bad for you. In moderation some do have positive effects.

Next to blood, naturally fermented wine is nature's most complex organic fluid. It contains over 300 different ingredients, more than half of which have only been discovered in the last 20 years. Naturally fermented wine boasts several different natural alcohols, sugars, enzymes and many minerals, as well as vitamins A, C and the B-complex – all in a form which many doctors claim is easily assimilated by the body.

A LITTLE WINE FOR YOUR HEALTH'S SAKE

The large number of enzymes which are responsible for each wine's distinctive flavour and character also make it an excellent drink for people who have difficulty absorbing nutrients – particularly fats – from food. And, according to many nutritionists, this group includes most people over the age of 40.

Vitamins and minerals, too, play an important part in the dietary virtues of good wine. Although wine contains only a small quantity of vitamin A, its B-complex content is high enough to make it a recommended source and its vitamin C content is also valuable. Its mineral composition includes calcium, magnesium, potassium and sulphur.

But a moderate amount of natural wine goes even further to support health. Anthocyanines, which have long been known to have an antibiotic effect against infection, are part of the pigmentation of grape skins and give wine its clear colour. Research shows that certain substances in wine are even capable of killing some of the detrimental micro-organisms which we consume with our food.

The French have always contended that wine stimulates the appetite, and research into this question at the University of California has confirmed the proverbial folk wisdom. The tannin content of wine, and its phenols and flavins (which are the source of wine's anaesthetic properties as well), all contribute to its positive effect on the appetite, particularly if you drink wine *before* your meal. Wine not only stimulates the appetite and starts the digestive juices flowing, but it also provides substances which then go on to encourage easy digestion and a more complete assimilation of food.

So, if you fancy it, take a little wine for your health's sake. The key to drinking wine for health lies in the word 'little'. Never feel that it is necessary to finish off a bottle of wine if this means that you will over-indulge. More than two or three glasses a day is simply too much.

MINIMIZE THE DAMAGE

Researchers now know that the effect of alcohol on one person will be quite different from its effect on another. There are no hard and fast rules about how much or how often you can drink and still 'get away with it'. But understanding more about alcohol and its effects can offer some protection from the long-term dangers of too much social drinking.

Not only do individual drinkers vary, but the effects of alcoholic beverages can vary as well, depending on various factors. There are some whose special properties you may well wish to avoid.

● **Beware of fizz** Studies on drinkers have demonstrated that alcohol consumed in a fizzy drink, such as champagne or whisky and soda, is absorbed much faster than when the alcohol is mixed with non-carbonated water or fruit juice.

Such findings also show that drinks with an alcohol content of 10–20 per cent are absorbed more rapidly than others when taken on an empty stomach. In a healthy person, this absorption is complete within 45 minutes to one-and-a-half hours. This means that a long whisky and water will make you feel higher than either a dry martini cocktail or a straight vodka.

● **The non-congenial congeners** The severity of hangovers varies considerably from one person to another. The worst hangovers result from drinking alcoholic beverages with the highest amounts of congeners – non-alcoholic substances left over from fermentation which give each drink its particular flavour.

Congeners are metabolized more slowly than alcohol itself, so they remain in the body longer, causing toxic effects. For some people, they cause allergic reactions. Champagne, brandy, gin and cheap wine all contain a high proportion of congeners; vodka and good, naturally fermented wine have far lower levels.

A QUICK GUIDE TO WINES AND YOUR BODY

There are roughly five classes of wine, each with its own characteristics, uses and drawbacks. The subtle differences between each, in terms of their different effects on your body, depend mostly on the variety of grapes used to make them, and on the soil and climate in which these grapes have been grown.

○ **The appetizer wines**
These wines contain 17–21 per cent alcohol. The group includes the rich, mellow sherries and the Madeiras. They boast more aromatic alcoholic substances, such as aldehydes and esters, than do table wines. This, say wine advocates, makes them valuable both as tranquillizers and stimulants – and from this point of view, the dryer and older the sherry the better. The appetizer wines also tend to have a lower total acidity than do table wines, but they are higher in calories.

○ **The sparkling wines**
Champagne is the best known of this group, which depend for their character on a carbon dioxide content under pressure of as much as 90 pounds per square inch (6.3 kg/sq cm). This gives them a double-edged reputation: they are both vivacious tonics and digestive disturbers.

Dry champagne is rich in sulphur and potassium, which some experts believe can play a role in detoxifying body wastes, as well as in protecting you against microbic and organic poisons. They recommend a glass or two before meals for those who are concerned about heart disease, since potassium salts contained in sparkling wine are believed to have a favourable influence on muscle tone, bringing better oxygenation to the heart and helping to strengthen the whole circulatory system. This is, however, an idea which is by no means universally accepted.

○ **The white table wines**
These wines have an alcohol content of 10–12 per cent alcohol and are most often recommended for people with digestive difficulty. Sweet wines from Anjou or Vouvray are believed to promote biliary secretions and stimulate the actions of the intestines. Sancerre, Rhine and Riesling wines are reputed to have diuretic properties, which is why they are often recommended for those who tend to have high blood pressure or who wish to lose weight. The experts say that most white wines are excellent for nervous stomachs.

○ **The red wines and rosés**
These also have an alcohol content of about 12 per cent and are rich in tannins, which are said to interact with vitamins and help increase the resistance of the capillary walls and retard their degeneration. Most red wines are used for their *tonic* properties. St Emilion is often prescribed for fatigue. Médoc is recommended for nervous depression. Red wines are also taken for fever and to counteract extreme weight loss.

○ **The dessert wines**
Port and dessert wines have an alcohol content of 18–21 per cent. Their sugar content is far too high to make them useful to anyone with a weight problem. The greatest recommendation for port seems to be its ability to induce sound sleep.

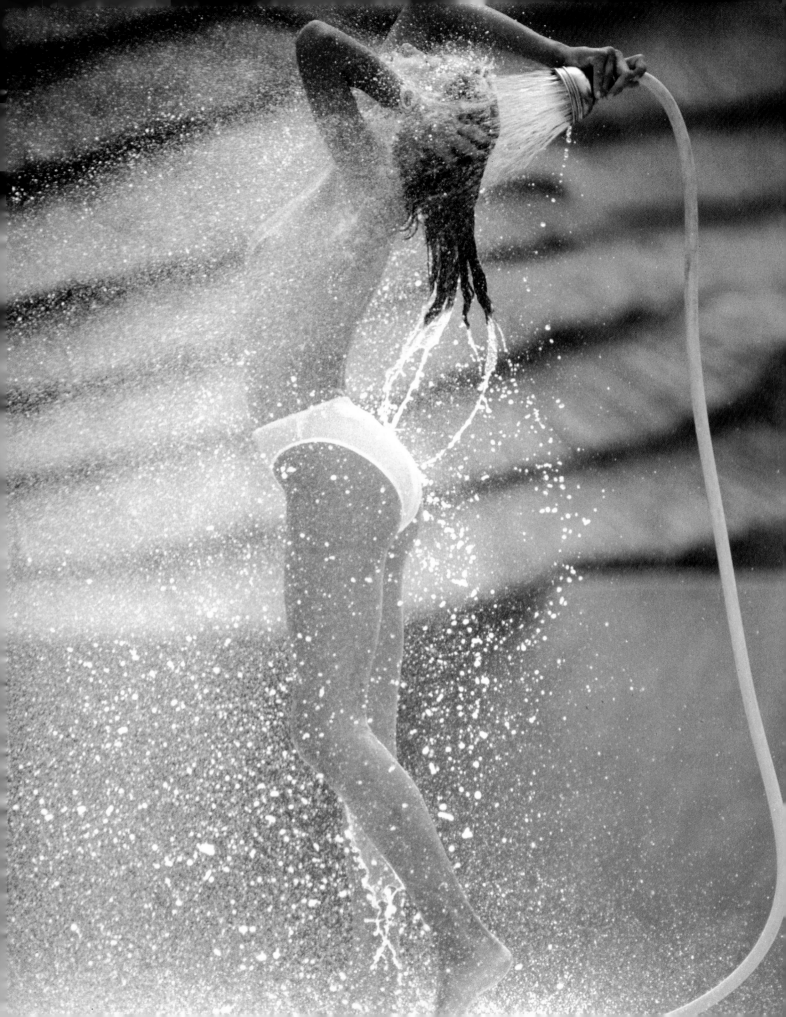

BODY TIME

Your body is the medium through which you experience reality. It is not – as our philosophical heritage from the Greeks would have us believe – an appendage to the soul. Far from it. How you perceive beauty, how you express love and creativity and intelligence, how you reason and think, even how you feel about yourself and your life are mediated through your body. To live fully your body needs to be fully alive.

Watch a young child running along the beach. Notice the fluid movements of his arms and legs and the way every movement seems to lead to the next without a break. Like a wild horse or a wolf he runs for the sheer pleasure of it. It feels good. Just as it feels good to us to laugh or make love. This is true aliveness – an aliveness which most of us lose not only because we don't exercise enough but also because the educational and religious tradition in which we have grown up does not fundamentally value this aliveness. It therefore makes little effort to preserve it. The physical training given in schools, like much of the exercise training handed out in fancy gyms and dance studios, tends to treat the body in a mechanical way – like some kind of dumb animal to be put through its paces without regard for how consciousness is connected with movement or how muscle tone and physical sensation can alter consciousness. As a result there are many of us who cannot feel fully alive in our bodies. We are carrying too little muscle or too much fat. We think of our bodies as objects and are far too critical about how they measure up against the current criteria for what is believed to be fashionable. We do not care for them lovingly – the way you would a precious child.

These forms of abuse or neglect, together with chronic muscle tension and flaccidity which result from lack of exercise or from exercising in a mechanical way, create in us a sense of numbness. It is a numbness so subtle that it is most often perceived (especially by women) as emotional rather than physical. It develops gradually, unnoticeably, until in time we lose much of our sensitivity and our capacity for experiencing pleasure from everyday things. In a sense, our bodies, which have gone unused, gradually die. That is the bad news. The good news is that, thanks to the dynamism of the human body, no matter how neglectful you have been a body can be resurrected from this living death. That is exactly what all of the 'body time' techniques, treats and treatments are designed to do – to re-establish the sense of aliveness of a healthy child and have you looking better than ever.

CONFRONT YOURSELF

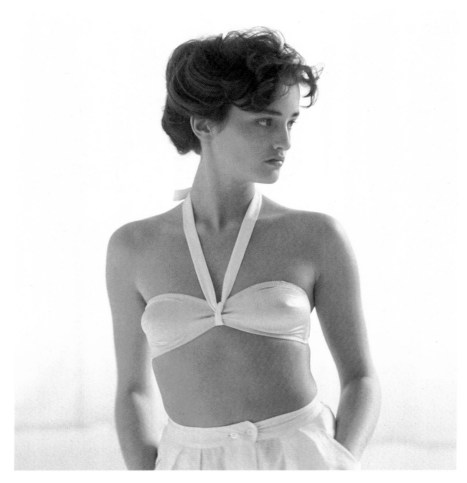

To make the most of your potential you truly have to *own* your body. This means realizing that your entire body, from the roots of your hair to the tips of your toes, is the embodiment of your *self*. Sadly, most of us dissociate ourselves from our bodies. We imagine ourself as a mind somewhere in our heads which is responsible for the rest of us from the neck down. This disassociation encourages us to treat our bodies with contempt: we eat the wrong foods, drink too much, worry too much and continually drive ourselves beyond the state of fatigue. Then, when we suffer from pains or get sick, we wonder foolishly why fate seems to have it in for us. Sound familiar?

Rather than treat your body like a machine which seems to break down for no apparent reason, you need to begin to listen to what it tells you. Very often we can prevent illness or heal ourselves by taking the trouble to tune into our bodies. By increasing your awareness and sensitivity throughout your body you can not only avoid many health and beauty hazards, you can also learn to apply all of yourself to whatever you are doing and

function at a much more efficient level in everything you do. More important, such *total* involvement can bring with it great joy and a sense of endless energy – energy that can transform your life.

It is important to begin by accepting your own form. All of us have things which we dislike about our bodies. It may be the size of your hips/waist/thighs, the shape of your nose or chin, your teeth, your hair, etc. We waste far too much time and energy worrying about the parts of ourselves which we dislike instead of focussing on the positive things and putting our energy into the task at hand. Try the following exercise to put your dislikes into perspective.

CONFRONT THE MIRROR

Stand in front of a full-length mirror and use a hand mirror to take a really good look at yourself from all angles. Make a list of all the things you dislike about yourself. Be thorough and write down everything you see which you dislike. Now take a pen and give each item a code. If it is something that cannot be changed,

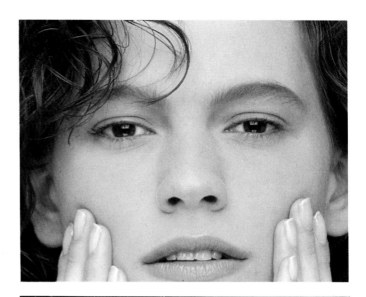

your height, for example, mark it with an 'I' for impossible. If it is something that would require professional help to fix, such as chipped or gappy teeth, bust size, disfiguring scars, mark it with a 'P'. If it is something which you know can be changed, such as your haircut, weight, excess body hair, mark it with a 'C'.

Now re-examine the list. First look at the 'Cs'. Decide whether you really care enough about the thing to change it. If you do, underline it and make a mental decision to take action on it. You will find helpful tips throughout the book which you can use to overcome these dislikes. If you don't care enough to do something about it, then it's not worth worrying about any more so cross it off your list. Now look at the 'Ps' and decide whether they are really a possibility. Could you afford the cost of professional help? Is the problem really that important to you? Again, either decide to do something about it and begin by making enquiries, or choose to accept it and cross it off your list. Finally, count the number of 'impossible' dislikes you are left with. Take another look at yourself in the mirror and, this time, beside the first list, make a second list of all the things you like about yourself. Go on writing things down until your list of likes is at least as long as your list of impossible dislikes. If you run out of things you like, then write down the things about yourself which you don't mind. Make a decision to begin to appreciate and accentuate your positive features and not to dwell on your dislikes. The more you focus on your good points the less you'll notice or even care about your dislikes .

REVEAL YOUR TRUE FORM

Number one on most people's lists are body shapes and sizes. Although we are stuck with our basic skeletal and muscular frame, for better or for worse, we can do a lot to improve the way we look, walk and feel. The secret to being happy in your body is not starving yourself to look like a lithe fashion model – most of us never will – but finding your own *true* form. This means losing excess weight, toning your muscles and improving your posture. We have both been amazed by how much the shapes of our bodies have improved through the changes we've made in our diet and through exercise. And it works for everybody. The most exciting thing is discovering, when your true form begins to emerge, that you actually like your natural shape after all.

SAMPLE LIST

I = impossible   P = professional   C = change

DISLIKES	CODE
○ Bust too small	I/P

I wouldn't want to go through implantation surgery. Perhaps if I slim a bit I'll lose some weight from my hips and my bust won't look so small by comparison.

○ **Hips too big**   C

I really would like to do something once and for all about my weight problem so that I can wear more attractive clothes and feel like less of a moose.

○ **Double chin**   C/P

A face lift would be too expensive. I'll look into exercises to tone my chin and neck muscles.

○ **Thin hair, bad cut**   C

It's definitely time to change this haircut. I think perhaps I'll try to get a better hairdresser, even if it's more expensive. Hopefully a good professional will be able to tell me what style would suit me best. Perhaps I'll look into the possibility of a perm or some highlights.

○ **Dark circles under eyes**   I/C

I'm not sure I can get rid of them. Perhaps a detoxification diet for a few days would help?

○ **Lopsided ears**   I

I think I'm stuck with this.

○ **Splitting nails**   C

I would really love to have long strong nails. I'll promise myself to manicure them regularly and take some supplements to strengthen them.

○ **Cellulite**   I/P/C

I'm not sure how to get rid of it, but I can't accept it so I'll do what I can.

○ **Hairy legs**   P

For the moment I don't really care, but perhaps I'll get my legs waxed before I go on holiday.

LIKES

○ **Eyes**

People have told me they're nice.

○ **Hands**

I quite like my hands.

○ **Hair**

I like the natural colour of my hair.

○ **Legs**

I suppose my legs aren't too bad, although I could lose some weight from my thighs.

Body Time

BODY SCULPTING

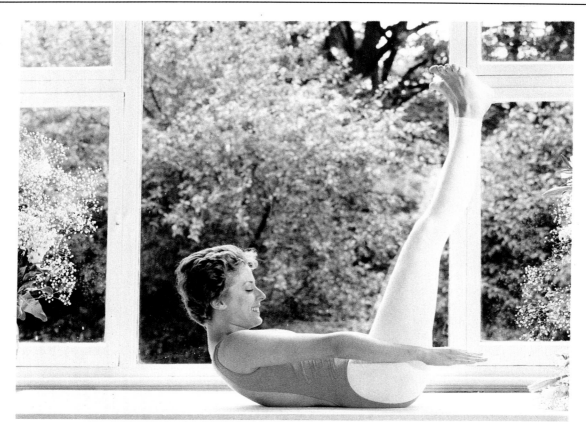

Michelangelo claimed that he never imposed any shape or form onto the piece of marble he was carving. Instead he simply used his sculptor's tools to *reveal the natural form hidden within* the marble. A neglected body is like his marble. Within it is hidden its vital, naturally healthy and lean form. We looked carefully at many forms of exercise from aerobic dancing to weight-training in our search for a method which would help us uncover it for us and others – a biological method of 'living sculpture'. And what we found was far removed from all the others. It's called Pilates and has been taught to us by Alan Herdman in his London studio.

The Pilates method was designed early on in the century by a German *émigré* called Joseph Pilates who himself was looking for a way of strengthening the body to enhance resistance to serious illness such as tuberculosis. It consists of a few carefully performed movements in sequence – mostly carried out on special equipment. The movements are slow and deliberate, each of them done with full mental awareness. These movements, carried out regularly two or three times a week, are capable not only of transforming the shape of the body but also of helping to bring mind and body together as a single dynamic whole. And there are only two or three other approaches to exercise we have ever seen that can also make this claim. The trouble with the classic Pilates exercises is that to do them you need to visit an exercise studio regularly – and one that is well equipped with all the special pulleys and ropes and moving tables.

Alan Herdman has taken the Pilates principles and worked them into a complete exercise routine which you can do three or four times a week without any special equipment at all – except perhaps a chair and a broom handle. The exercises are simple and superb. Six weeks on them makes you rediscover that sense of aliveness which belongs to the running child. They are well worth the effort.

But remember, each and every one of these exercises is designed to be done with awareness, not mechanically as most people are taught to do callisthenics. The breathing is important too. You always breathe out during the part of the exercise when your body is making the effort. This helps keep an easy flow of movement, makes your movements more co-ordinated, and eliminates tensions. Your breath should be light but not shallow. Be sure to use your lungs rather than your stomach and diaphragm. The length of time you spend on a movement and your breathing in or out should match.

THE HUNDRED

● **Bonuses** This exercise is excellent for strengthening the muscles of the stomach and lower back and can be a great help to women who suffer from period cramps. It also improves lung capacity.

● **Here's how** Lie with your back completely flat on the floor with your arms raised towards the ceiling and your knees bent up to your chest. Pull your navel towards your back, elongating your spine and relaxing your shoulders. Breathe in and lift your head and shoulders off the floor, with your chin pulled down towards your chest. Check that the base of your spine is firmly on the floor. Breathe out, stretching your arms down to your sides and taking your legs out to an angle of 60 degrees. Turn out (rotate) your legs from the hip joint and flex your feet, squeezing the backs of your thighs and your inner thighs together. Remember to keep your chin down to your chest and continue to pull your navel towards your spine. Holding this position, breathe in through your nose for 5 seconds and breathe out through your mouth for 5 seconds, gently beating time with your hands. Keep your shoulders down and your arms stretched beyond your hips. Do this ten times. Then return to starting position. Rest, holding onto your knees and pulling them gently into your chest.

SIDE LIFT

● **Bonuses** This exercise firms the muscles of the waist and stomach and strengthens muscles in the hip area.

● **Here's how** Lie on your right side with your back against a wall to give you extra support. Keeping your body in a straight line, extend your right arm on the floor above your head, rest your head on the arm and press the palm of your hand to the floor. Squeeze your legs together and stretch away from your centre. Pull in your stomach muscles back towards the wall. Bend the top arm to support your torso by placing it on the floor approximately 6 inches (15cm) in front of the breastbone. Breathing out, pull in your stomach muscles and lift both legs off the floor as high as possible, keeping your feet together. Breathing in slowly, lower them to the floor. Repeat ten times on each side.

● **Variation** Using the same starting position, lift both legs as before. When your legs are raised as high as possible, continue to lift the top leg, keeping your bottom leg suspended. Lower your top leg slowly towards the bottom one and take them both down to the floor. Always breathe out to raise and in to lower. Repeat ten times on each side.

opposite **The Hundred**
top **Side Lift**
bottom **Side Lift variation**

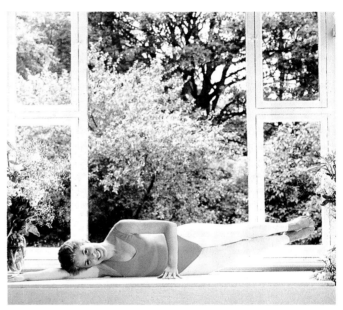

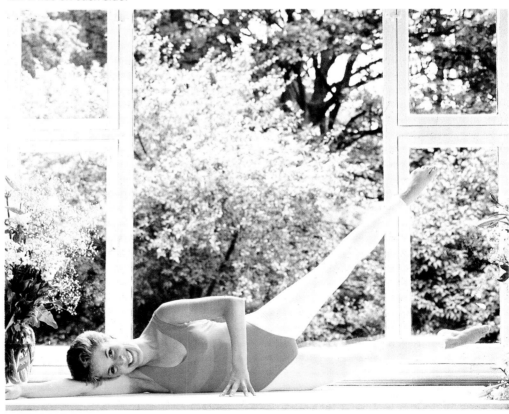

Body Time

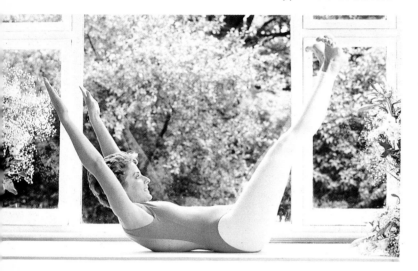

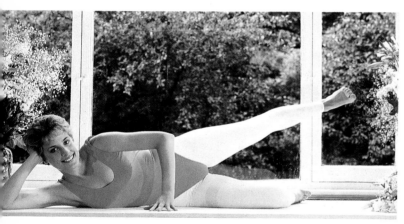

top **Double Leg Stretch**
middle **Leg Lift 1**
bottom **Leg Lift 2**
opposite **Side Stretch**

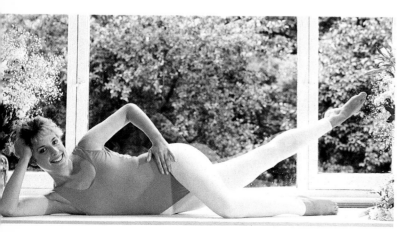

DOUBLE LEG STRETCH

● **Bonuses** This exercise increases the mobility in the shoulders and upper back, firms stomach muscles and helps lower back problems.

● **Here's how** Lie on your back and bend your knees up towards your chest, shoulder-width apart. Hold the outside of your knees lightly, elongating your neck, relaxing your shoulders, pulling your navel towards your spine and pressing your tailbone to the floor. Without moving your knees, pull your head and shoulders up and press your chin to your chest, keeping your navel pressed towards your spine. Breathing in, stretch out your arms and legs to an angle of 60 degrees. As they straighten, flex your feet and turn out (rotate) your legs from the hip joint, squeezing your inner thighs together. Breathing out, stretch your arms up to the ceiling and back behind your head, brushing your ears with the inside of your arms as they pass. At the fullest stretch of your arms, pull in your stomach more. Breathing in, move your arms in a wide arc to each side and up towards your toes. Reach your hands towards your feet and slowly point your toes. Breathing out slowly, bend your knees and elbows, grasp your knees and return to starting position. Repeat ten times.

SIDE STRETCH

● **Bonuses** This exercise tones the upper arms and slims the waist.

● **Here's how** Sitting astride a dining chair with your back straight and your navel pulled towards your spine, make sure that your neck and shoulders are relaxed. Place your feet firmly on the floor with the inside of your thighs gently gripping the chair. Use your left hand to hold the back of the chair. Breathing in, reach your right hand to the ceiling, feeling a stretch from hip to fingers. Breathing out, curve and stretch your right side over to the left, keeping the right hip pressed firmly down towards the chair. Breathing in slowly, return to the centre, re-establishing the starting position. Change your arm and stretch to the other side. Repeat five times to each side.

LEG LIFT 1

● **Bonuses** This exercise tones the outer thighs and helps firm the bottom. It is also good for the waistline.

● **Here's how** Lie on your right side in a straight line with your right arm stretched out on the floor above your head. Bend your elbow and rest your head in your hand. Bend your left arm and place your left hand on your left hip, pushing down gently to keep your waist long. Now bend your right leg to a comfortable angle keeping your spine very straight and your foot flexed. Breathing out, lift your top leg approximately 8 inches (20 cm) higher than your hip. Breathing in slowly, lower your leg gently to the floor. Repeat ten times on each side.

LEG LIFT 2

● **Bonuses** This exercise strengthens the muscles of the inner thigh, firms the thighs and increases mobility in the hips.

● **Here's how** Lie on your right side in a straight line with your right arm extended on the floor above your head. Bend your elbow and rest your head in your hand. Bend your left arm in front of the chest with your hand on the floor supporting your torso. Bend your left leg forwards and rest it on the floor in a comfortable position with your spine very straight and your foot pointed. Breathe out, lifting your bottom leg as high as possible. Breathe in, lowering the bottom leg slowly to the floor. Repeat ten times on each side.

LEG LIFT 3
⬤ **Bonuses** This exercise firms and slims the bottom and stretches the hamstrings.

⬤ **Here's how** Lying on your right side in a straight line, bend your right arm and rest your head on your hand. Bend your left arm in front of your chest, placing your hand on the floor to support your torso. Now bend your right knee into a comfortable angle, keeping your spine very straight and your foot flexed. Breathing out, lift your leg to hip level, pulling your navel towards the spine, and swing your leg slowly forwards to an angle of 90 degrees. Lift your leg up approximately 6 inches (15 cm). Breathing in, lower your leg 6 inches (15 cm) and return to the starting position. Repeat ten times on each side.

SQUEEZES
⬤ **Bonuses** This exercise firms the inner thighs and the stomach muscles.

⬤ **Here's how** Lying on your back on the floor with your arms relaxed and your knees bent, place your feet together, soles flat on the floor. Keeping your feet together, open your knees and place a cushion firmly between them. Breathing out, slowly squeeze the cushion with the inside of your thighs, counting 8 seconds. As the cushion is squeezed, press the base of your spine into the floor, relaxing your neck and shoulders and pulling your navel into the spine. Breathing in slowly, relax the knees and inner thighs. Repeat ten times.

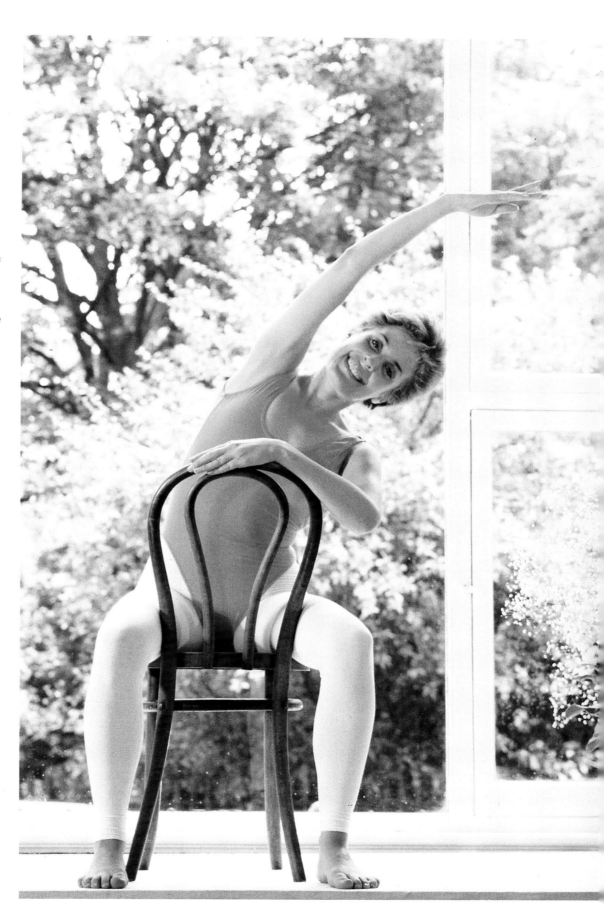

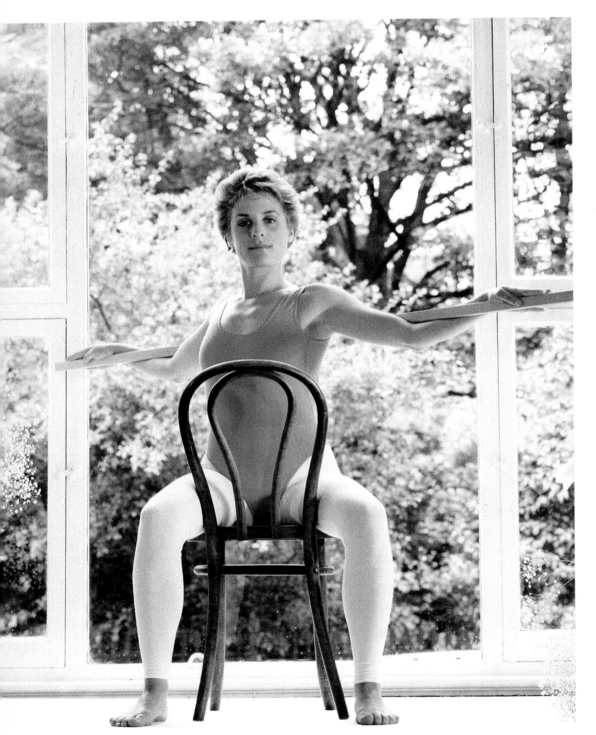

LEG LIFT 4

● **Bonuses** These exercises firm the backs of thighs and the buttocks.

● **Here's how** Lying on your stomach on the floor with your arms bent and the palms of your hands flat on the floor, rest your forehead on the backs of your hands. Now, with your legs straight and rotated outwards from the hip joints and your buttocks pulled together, place your feet about 8 inches (20 cm) apart and point your toes. Pull your stomach muscles away from the floor to support your back. Breathing out, tighten the backs of your thighs and lift your right leg 4 inches (10 cm) off the floor. Breathe in and lower it to the floor. Repeat eight times with each leg.

LEG LIFT 5

● **Here's how** Keeping your feet in the same position as in Leg Lift 4, stretch your arms out until they are straight and your hands are in line with your feet (about shoulder-width apart). Support your lower back by pulling your stomach muscles up and lift your head, hands and feet 2 inches (5 cm) off the floor. Breathing out, beat your legs together sixteen times. Rest, breathing in. Repeat four times.

POLE SWING

● **Bonuses** This exercise loosens the shoulder girdle and relieves tension in the upper back and between the

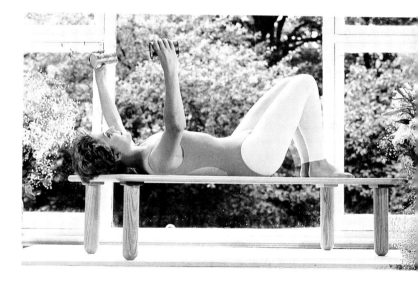

shoulder-blades.

● **Here's how** Sitting astride a dining chair with your back straight and your navel pulled towards your spine, relax your neck and shoulders and place your feet firmly on the floor with the inside of your thighs gently gripping the chair. Place a pole (a broomstick will do) across your shoulder-blades approximately level with your breastbone, wrapping your arms over the pole so that your hands are in front of it. Keeping your spine straight and your head still, swing the pole from side to side breathing freely.

FLIES 1

● **Bonuses** This firms the underarms and opens the upper chest, toning up the pectorals and improving the look of the breasts.

● **Here's how** Lying on your back on a flat surface, such as a bench, off of the floor, bend your knees and press your feet and knees gently together. Pull your navel towards the spine. Holding onto soup tins, straighten your arms up to 90 degrees. With the tins touching, curve your arms outwards to form a circle. Breathing out, open your arms into a wide half circle. Breathing in, close your arms. Do this eight times opening your arms with the outward breath and eight times opening them with the inward breath.

FLIES 2

● **Bonuses** This exercise is

good for the bust, the chest, the triceps and the inside arms.

● **Here's how** With your head at the edge of the bench and your torso and legs in the same position as in Flies 1, hold one tin with both hands and straighten your arms to 90 degrees. Bend your elbows outwards, forming a diamond shape. Holding this shape and breathing out, pull it slowly back behind your head as far as possible. Breathing in, pull your arms back through the centre and downwards towards the navel. Do this eight times with the outward breath on the stretch and eight times with the inward breath on the stretch.

FLIES 3

● **Bonuses** This exercise is good for the chest, triceps and underarms.

● **Here's how** Sitting up straight on a chair, stomach muscles supporting your lower back and with your feet planted firmly on the ground, put a soup tin in your right hand and raise it towards the ceiling, keeping your arm straight. Support your working arm with the left hand. Now slowly lower the tin behind your head, still keeping your arm straight while breathing in, making sure you keep your elbow by your ear. Raise it slowly to the starting position on the out-breath and begin again. (The work is on the raise.) Do this eight times, then change arms and repeat.

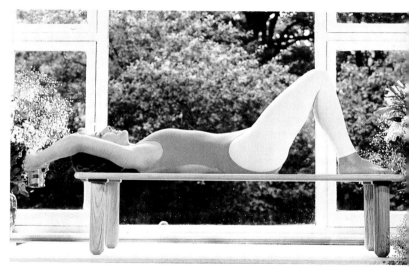

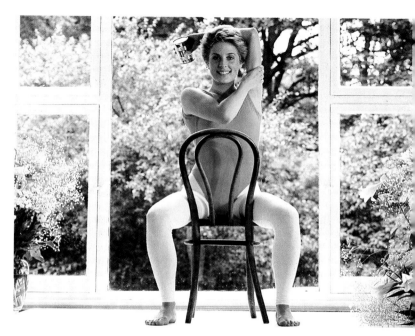

FAT BANISHING

Trying to shed fat can seem an enormous challenge. For some it means constant self-abnegation and is a kind of continual battle with guilt and over-indulgence. For others it is a source of constant frustration. There is no question that if you are serious about shedding excess fat and keeping it off you will need to change not only your diet but also your life style. You'll need to make sure you have time and skills for deep relaxation instead of turning to food for solace and you'll need gradually to work your way into a programme of active exercise which gets your heart and lungs working for 45 minutes at a time at least four times a week. The one thing you can forget is calorie counting. It simply doesn't work. At least not long term. This is something both of us know from experience as well as from combing the slimming literature in search of answers. What *does* work is, first, a lot more activity and, second, learning to combine your food properly.

Getting more exercise doesn't mean killing yourself in a strenuous aerobics class or training for your first marathon. It means becoming more active in the way you lead your life. For instance, when you arrive at a building where there is a lift and you are going to the fourth floor, take the stairs instead. While you are sitting in front of the television in the evening, do some slow stretching exercises. Or whenever you have the chance to be active, take it. Soon this will become almost second nature to you. By then you will find your metabolism is working better and you don't suffer from that sluggish feeling which makes many of us eat too much and get fat. It also means getting out every day, winter and summer, wet or not, and walking briskly for at least 30, and preferably 45, minutes.

NATURAL AID FOR SLIMMING

The essential free amino acid phenylalanine is a natural appetite suppressant for six out of ten people. It can be helpful for people just beginning to food combine (see p. 94) until their false hunger disappears. It appears to have a number of other therapeutic properties as well – from acting as an anti-depressant to helping eliminate the chronic pain of arthritis and back injuries. Phenylalanine needs to be taken on an empty stomach together with vitamin B6 and vitamin C, which are needed for its conversion. It appears to work to reduce hunger in various ways. It is converted into noradrenaline in the body. Noradrenaline is an important brain chemical – an excitatory neurotransmitter which elevates your mood and quite simply makes you feel like eating less. Amphetamines – the prescription drugs used to suppress appetite – also work to release noradrenaline in the brain and to block its reabsorption. The trouble is that with amphetamines you quickly build up a tolerance to them so they cease to be effective and you need to take ever-increasing doses to get the desired effect. Amphetamines also have dangerous side-effects when taken over a period of time. Amongst other things, they force your body to produce more noradrenaline than is its wont without supplying the raw materials from which it can be made. This can lead to a deficiency of this important neurotransmitter.

Phenylalanine is different and it is safe. It normalizes brain and nerve levels of noradrenaline, suppressing appetite and making you feel energetic and positive without dangerous side-effects or the problem of building up tolerance. Phenylalanine appears to be important in another way too. According to recent research, the hypothalamus is the control centre for a chemical called cholecystokin – CCK – which is made in the brain and the intestines and is believed to be important in giving you either a feeling of hunger or of satiety. Too much CCK appears to make people undereat while too little encourages gluttony. Phenylalanine availability has been linked to CCK production through noradrenaline, since high levels of this neurotransmitter in the brain can spur the release of CCK which in turn reduces appetite.

Phenylalanine comes in various forms. The kind used for appetite control is usually L-phenylalanine or DL- phenylalanine – which is also used for the control of chronic pain. It is usually taken with B6 and vitamin C first thing in the morning in 500 mg capsules, since they are more readily absorbed than tablets. The one caution about its use is in the case of someone with high blood pressure since this amino acid can heighten blood pressure if used in too high a dose. As with any of the accessory nutrients it is wise to consult a nutritionally aware physician before embarking on a course of them.

AMINO FAT-BURNER FOR SUSTAINED ENERGY

L-carnitine is another amino acid currently attracting a lot of attention as a means of encouraging weight loss. Not an essential amino acid, L-carnitine can be made in

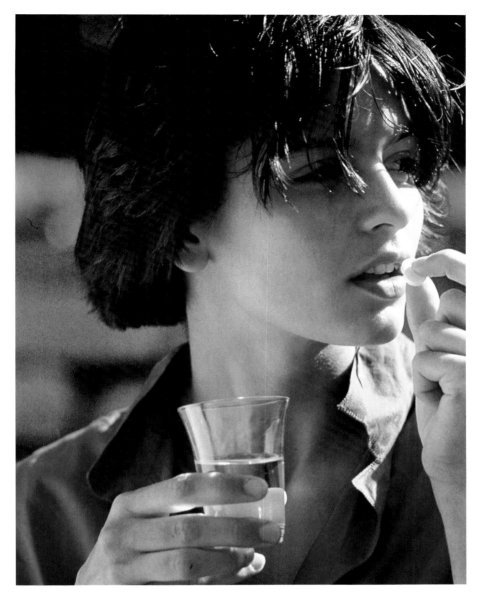

the liver from two other amino acids – lysine and methionine – in the presence of vitamins C, B6, niacin and iron. It is used in your body as a substance which transfers fatty acids through the membranes of the mitochondria – the body's minute energy factories in each cell – so that they can be burnt and turned into energy. If not enough carnitine is available, then fatty acids are not metabolized well. This can lead to a build-up of fat stored in the body as well as to high blood fats. Supplements of L-carnitine have been shown in animal experiments to improve fat metabolism, reduce blood cholesterol and triglyceride levels and lower blood pressure. Also, in experiments on animals, this free amino is currently attracting interest because of its ability to prolong a creature's average lifespan, probably because it enhances the anti-oxidant effects of other nutrients such as vitamin E and vitamin C by carrying them to the mitochondria where the aging free radicals

are generated. L-carnitine is also being widely used as a supplement for athletes – one to two 250 mg capsules a day – because it enhances the body's ability to burn fat for energy and therefore prolongs endurance. It can sometimes be helpful for weight loss because of this ability and because it also protects the body from ketosis – a common problem for many people on weight-reducing diets. Ketosis means an accumulation of fat waste products called ketones or ketone bodies. This build-up tends to make the blood acidic and leads to the loss of potassium, calcium and magnesium from the body. It can cause kidney damage and even be life-threatening if it goes uncontrolled. Carnitine supple-mentation can prevent this. L-carnitine is believed to be the best form of this amino acid for it is the most active and doesn't cause muscle weakness as can the D- and the DL- forms. It is generally given on an empty stomach – from 250 mg to 500 mg two or three times a day.

FOOD COMBINING

One of us (Leslie) tends to gain weight easily even on the best of diets, partly because of a great passion for food and the over-indulgence which goes with it, partly because of the way her metabolism works – slowly – despite her taking a lot of regular exercise.

Since beginning to practise the art of conscientious food combining with a high-raw diet, things have been so much easier for her that it is hard to remember the way they were before. We've found that food combining is great in other ways, too. It helps ward off a tendency to get colds and other minor ailments. And it protects against the build-up of cellulite.

The old days of meat and potatoes are something you want to leave behind. Concentrated protein foods such as nuts, seeds, dairy products, eggs and flesh foods need an acid medium for efficient digestion, while concentrated starches such as beans and grains, potatoes, breads, cereals, yams and pumpkins need an alkaline one. Mixing these foods delays digestion, tends to produce toxicity in the system and can be responsible both for increasing appetite and causing digestive upsets. What you can get away with is the occasional garnish of protein foods or fruit foods – such as sesame seeds or raisins – in a dish to which you would never normally add them in greater quantity.

Fruit passes through your digestive system very rapidly and requires little action by digestive enzymes in order to break it down for body use. If fruit is eaten at a meal with other foods, its digestion and assimilation will be slowed drastically and you can get fermentation in the gut. This results in indigestion, wind and discomfort. In some people fruits eaten this way can turn into alcohol in the stomach which can then affect mind and mood.

Breakfast should be an entirely fruit meal. You can eat as much as you like. Your liver – the body's most important organ for detoxification – is most active between midnight and midday. Eating fruit, unlike taking in starch or protein foods, allows this detoxification process to continue unimpeded. All other foods interfere with it. You may have more fruit mid-morning if you still feel hungry.

● **Go for a salad meal once a day** A beautiful fresh salad based on home-grown or store-bought sprouted seeds and grains is the mainstay of high-energy food combining. Making one of your meals each day a huge salad of fresh, crisp vegetables is the best possible way to get optimal support for rebuilding cells and tissues, rebalancing biochemical processes and restoring normal metabolism.

● **Steer clear of chemical additives** Foods which have been excessively processed to alter their natural state (such as white breads, sugar, most meats, sweets, coffee and most of the ready-in-a-minute convenience foods) are depleted of nutrients and tend to contain potentially harmful additives.

Whole grains and cooked vegetables, legumes and dairy products, fresh fish, poultry and game are delicious and satisfying. They are good sources of sustained energy (particularly the grains) and useful as providers of proteins for the body's amino acid pool. Serve them as side dishes at your meals.

Your body, like the earth itself, is 70 per cent water, so 70 per cent of what you eat each day needs to be chosen from the high-water foods: fresh fruits and vegetables eaten raw. But there may be days when you find you have eaten more of the heavier foods than you should because of being invited out or having to eat in restaurants. Then it is a good idea to make the next day an all-raw day.

Your digestive system needs time to complete the digestion of a meal before you put anything else into it. Four or five hours must elapse between lunch and dinner, otherwise digestion is not complete and increased toxicity can ensue. Do drink spring water or herb tea between meals if you like, and if a meal is delayed beyond four or five hours after your last meal you can have a piece or two of fruit to tide you over.

● **Don't mix foods that fight** At first glance the chart opposite may seem complicated. It isn't really. It is all a matter of getting the basic principles right. Eat fruit on its own or at least 20 minutes (in the case of bananas, 45 minutes) before a meal. Keep your concentrated proteins (such as chicken or fish) separate from starches (such as potatoes or rice). You'll notice that some of the fruits combine better than others, but don't become neurotic about it. Two weeks of food combining will get you well into the swing of things so that you rarely have to bother even looking at the chart. And you can eat as much as you like provided you chew well and listen carefully to the dictates of your own appetite. The greatest wisdom of all for health and vitality comes from within.

Body Time

94

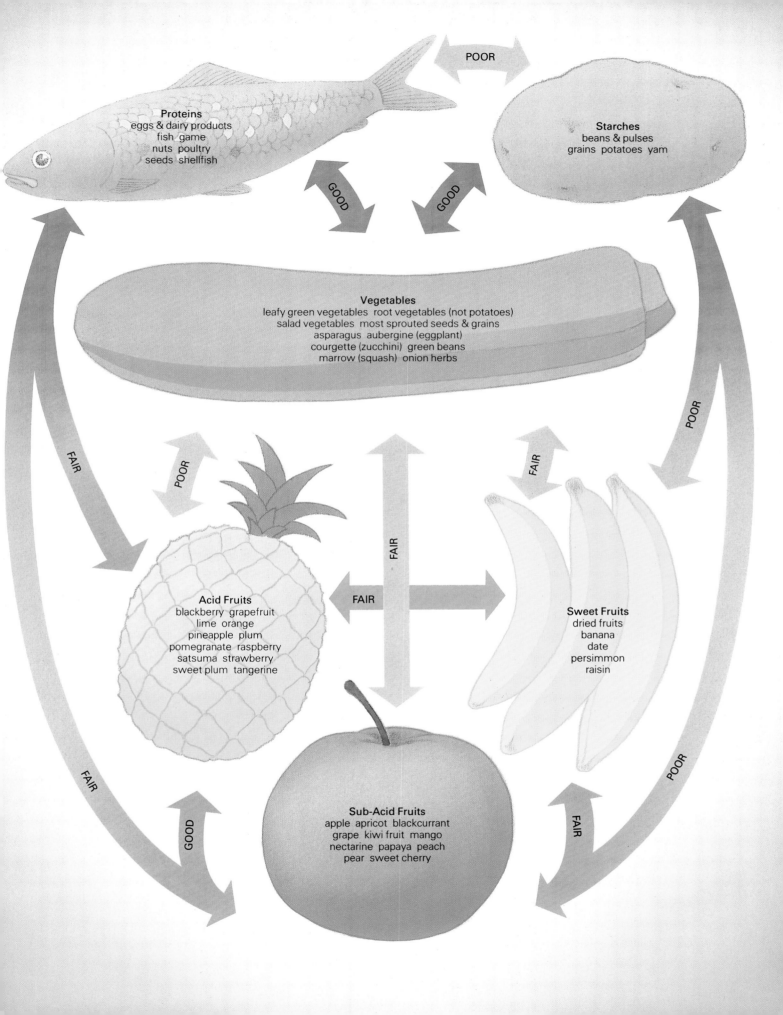

THIN THIGHS

Many British and American doctors insist that cellulite doesn't exist. We find this attitude hard to believe considering the serious work their European colleagues have done defining the condition and measuring the effectiveness of various approaches to treat this common problem.

These scientists have discovered that cellulite tends to begin when your body is undergoing dramatic hormonal changes such as in puberty, during pregnancy and at the first sign of menopause or if you start taking the birth control pill. Some have highlighted the relationship between the development of cellulite and general toxicity in the body. The woman who is unable to eliminate toxic wastes efficiently from her system, or whose diet and inability to cope with stress produce more metabolic wastes than her system can cope with, falls prey to the problem. Others have pointed out the correlation between poor circulation or inadequate lymphatic drainage in the body and the development of cellulite. Women with cellulite also often have constipation, and an underactive thyroid or poor liver function or both.

CHANGE THE WAY YOU EAT
The internal pollution problems which encourage cellulite are made worse by certain foods and drinks. Any woman serious about ridding her body of cellulite needs to avoid them. They include prepared and smoked fish and meats such as ham, bacon and sausages; refined carbohydrates and processed foods, with all their additives; salted foods, alcohol and coffee. Cigarette smoking is also a bad thing, since nicotine not only interferes with circulation and the oxygenation of cells, but also because other chemicals in cigarette smoke, such as acetaldehyde, are potent destroyers of the nutrients your body needs to protect collagen fibres from crosslinking and to keep capillaries strong and healthy.

But these are just the negatives. Food can be used against cellulite in a positive way too. A high-raw diet and conscientious food combining can be an enormous help in eliminating cellulite. The fibre in such a diet plays a large part in this kind of detoxification as well.

FABULOUS FIBRE
Dietary fibre is something which we have heard a lot about lately. Women are constantly being urged to eat bran (the only kind of fibre most doctors seem to have

heard of). It is supposed to help keep you thin and unconstipated, thanks to all the cellulose it contains. However, dietary fibre is not just made up of cellulose. There are other constituents of fibre which appear to be more important than cellulose when it comes to detoxification and protection against internal pollution and which are particularly useful in combatting cellulite. These include water-soluble hemicellulose, pectins, gums, mucilages and lignin – all of which are found in great quantity in fresh vegetables and fruits. Any anticellulite regime should be high in these raw foods.

SUPPLEMENTAL HELP
There are a number of nutritional supplements which can form a part of a total body approach to fighting cellulite. They include minerals such as iodine, which are found in sea plants, ascorbic acid, zinc, and the bioflavonoids as well as some of the B vitamins, particularly vitamin B3, which encourages circulation, and B6, which is a natural diuretic. Herbs such as alfalfa, dandelion and cornsilk make excellent, mildly diuretic tisanes.

SKIN-BRUSHING IS A KEY
A simple technique called skin-brushing can lend great help in banishing cellulite. Spend 5 minutes a day, before your bath, brushing your skin all over with a natural fibre brush. Begin at the top of the shoulders and cover the whole body (not the head) with long, smooth strokes over shoulders, arms and trunk in a downward motion. You need only cover your skin once for it to work. How firmly you press depends entirely on how toned your skin and body are already, so go easy to begin with. Almost one-third of the body's waste products can be eliminated through the skin, so a skin that is brushed regularly yields up the most amazing quantity of rubbish which would otherwise remain in the body to interfere with cellular metabolism and produce unsightly pockets of cellulite. If you brush your skin all over for 3 to 5 minutes and then take a damp flannel and wipe it over your body before you bathe, after a few days the smell of the flannel will be quite revolting because of the waste products that have come directly through the skin's surface.

The action that skin-brushing has on the lymphatic system of the body is even more important in keeping cellulite at bay. Unlike the circulation of the blood, which

Body Time

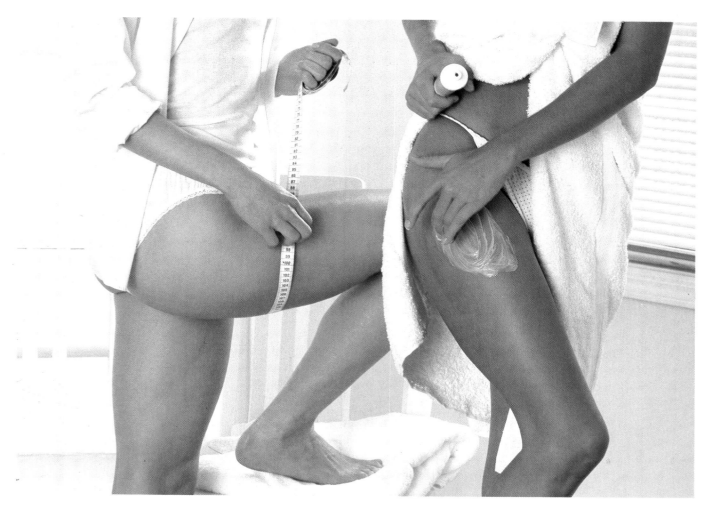

is controlled by the pumping of the heart, the lymphatic system has no pump. It is the normal contraction and relaxation of muscles in the body and the force of gravity which act to propel the lymph back through its channels and eliminate the wastes it has gathered.

Because of the stimulating action on the tissues beneath the skin, regular skin-brushing encourages efficient lymphatic drainage and is an extraordinarily effective technique for cleansing the lymphatic system.

CREAMS AND POTIONS HELP

European manufacturers have now produced creams which are designed specifically to alter cellulite-related changes in the skin tissue and help reduce cellulite areas. You rub them on your skin and they work by gently stimulating circulation to help eliminate the build-up of metabolic wastes and to drain subcutaneous tissue. And while none of the locally applied products and salon treatments for cellulite are going to yield much benefit on their own, together with the right kind of diet, nutritional supplements and skin-brushing they can go a long way towards banishing those unsightly lumps and bumps on thighs and hips for ever.

Massage can also help. It improves circulation in the localized cellulite areas, it helps bring wastes to the surface of the skin and it physically helps to break down the gel-filled pockets of cellulite, dispersing them. Massage should be done in a definite way before your bath: begin with effleurage, a light stroking movement on the surface of the skin, always stroking towards the heart. Then take hold of your flesh with both hands and, pulling it away from the bone, squeeze it as you would knead bread, first with one hand and then with the other. Then make a fist with both hands, pushing your knuckles deep into the cellulite areas, twisting them in a circular motion at the same time, for not more than 3 or 4 minutes at a time in one area. This movement, more than any other, helps to break up the deposits of cellulite and disperse them, but you have to work up to it each time. Finally, return to the soft stroking you began with. This routine should be done four or five times a week. You will notice that the cellulite seems to get worse as the water pockets beneath the skin begin to respond to pressures and become more sensitive to touch. But this reaction, which usually takes place between a week and two weeks after the treatment begins, is only a prelude to its ultimate dispersal.

BEAUTY AND THE BREAST

Your breasts need special treatment for them to remain firm and well contoured. This is because the breast is physiologically quite different from any other part of a woman's body. It consists of a gland surrounded by fat cells and connective tissue in which there is a rich supply of blood vessels and lymphatics and on which its size and shape largely depend, but which is completely lacking in muscle. Neither is it fixed to the chest. Instead, the breasts are suspended from a fan of skin that extends downwards from the neck and acts like a natural bra to support them. If this skin becomes loose, if the circulation to the underlying tissue is poor or if hydration is decreased from, say, too much exposure to the sun, then breasts lose their natural size and firmness and begin to sag.

FIRM AND SHAPELY

The time to begin caring for breasts is long before you have any reason to worry – by making sure your daily routine includes the things which keep them firm and shapely, such as hydrotherapy and specific exercise movements for the underlying musculature. Occasional cosmetic 'cures' both in salons and at home can help too. So can maintaining a steady body weight, since yo-yoing up and down on slimming diets or any kind of rapid weight gain or loss, even if it happens only once in a lifetime, is a sure way to ruin the look and firmness of your breasts.

BUY A GOOD BRA

A bra which is not properly fitted can also do a lot of damage. Too tight it can interfere with the circulation of the blood. Wearing a bra too loose, or no bra at all, particularly when you are exercising or moving about vigorously, can lead to a gradual breakdown of tissue firmness too, whatever your political views on going braless may be. That is why French women, who are the most knowledgeable in the world about how to care for their breasts (and the most obsessed) tend, except for when for the sake of fashion they *must* go braless, to wear a bra at all times. For a good bra, fitted to your body by an expert, is one of the best investments you can make for the future of your bust. Cotton is the best material because it allows air to penetrate easily and because it readily absorbs any perspiration given off by your body. It allows your skin to breathe.

THE WATER TREATMENT

Alternating applications of hot and cold water are worth more than the most expensive cosmetic products in protecting the firmness, smoothness and beauty of your bust. Take two basins of water, one hot and the other cold, each of which has a flannel in it. Then, wringing out the hot flannel, apply it to one breast and leave it there until the tissue is well warmed (usually 10–20 seconds). Now follow that with a cold compress on the same breast, doing one side at a time – three applications of hot and three of cold, always ending with the cold. Cold water on its own is the most effective medium for treating breasts which are losing their firmness and shape. Apply it with a spray, leaning over the sink, or after you have had a hot shower before getting out, by spraying in a circular motion around one breast and then the other in a figure-of-eight pattern, avoiding the nipple itself as much as you can.

BRUSH-UP FOR BUST BEAUTY

A dry brushing of the skin around the breasts, under the arms, on the neck and *décolletage* (which incidentally should also be lavishly covered with whatever breast cream, ampoule or oil you put on your bust) with a medium-firm natural bristle brush is another daily treatment which acts both as a preventative treatment against loss of shape and firmness and as a restorative one. Use movements which are circular from the inside towards the outside and continue until the skin slightly reddens. You should never irritate breast tissues or massage them. Massage can actually cause a loss in firmness. After such a dry brushing your skin will be highly receptive to whatever you put on it. Make this part of a daily routine, say, just before bath or shower, then, as you emerge, apply an oil, cream or lotion.

EXERCISE HOLDS A KEY

While exercise can do little to improve firmness and elasticity of connective tissue or circulation it can add support to the breasts by strengthening the pectoral muscles which underlie them, and the muscles of the neck to which the fan of skin from which they are suspended is attached. Exercise can also improve your posture – which is one of the most important factors of all when considering the look of your bust. In fact, there are some simple movements which will strengthen the

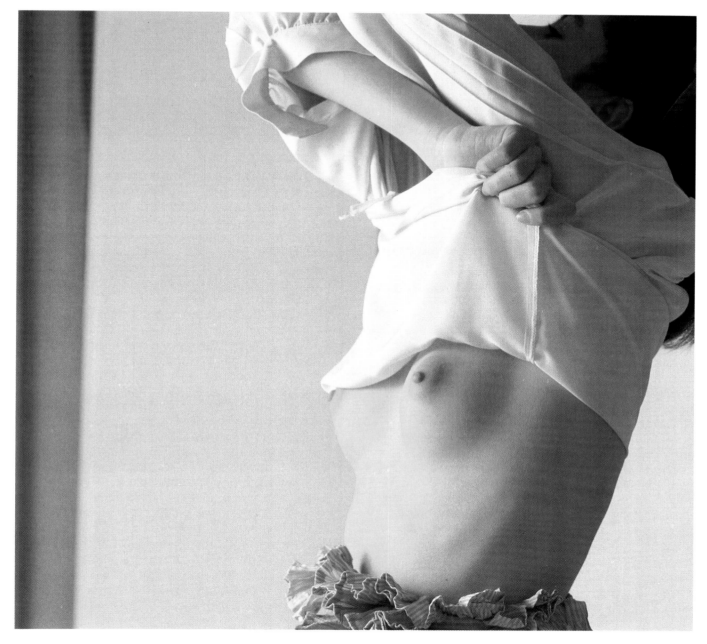

pectorals and improve the postural carriage of the upper body at the same time since they can affect the muscles of the neck and upper back too:

● **The Seagull** Holding your arms out to your sides at shoulder height with palms up, pivot your arms so that your palms are again upwards. All the while, be careful to keep your torso upright and still. Repeat the movement as many times as you can comfortably without feeling that your arms are dropping off, always in a slow rhythmical way.

● **Great Circles** Sitting erect in a straight chair with your hands on your knees, raise them to the sides, then high above your head, each forming a half circle. Now lower and raise them again in steady rhythm as many times as you comfortably can.

● **Between Heaven and Earth** Sitting again with a straight back, raise your arms above your head and grasp your fingers together so that each hand forms a hook for the other. Now pull outwards towards the sides, keeping your arms straight (elbows locked) and high above your head. Relax the pressure then pull again at least ten times, holding for 3 to 5 seconds each time.

● **The Grimace** Standing in front of a mirror, smile as widely as you possibly can while keeping your teeth together. You will see the musculature of your neck tighten and feel the way the muscles lift your bust. The more regularly you practise all four of these exercises (every day before a shower or bath) the more rapidly you will see the lift that exercise can bring to your bust.

Body Time

99

BE A BAT

They call it inversion therapy – a fancy modern name for an ancient and highly useful practice – hanging upside down. Yogis traditionally practise it in two forms – *sirsasana* (the head balance) and *sarvangasana* (the shoulder balance). Both are prized for their ability to keep the body young, healthy and full of vigour. We believe that regularly hanging upside down can make you feel and look terrific. It is good for your skin, the thyroid, the brain, the circulation and the posture. In addition, it benefits your spine, hips, knees and ankle joints and can be useful for improving muscle tone and for strengthening the spine. It also improves the circulation of the blood and lymphatic drainage, can relieve areas of chronic tension and static muscle fatigue in the body and even eliminate blocked sinuses. Sounds magic? In a sense, reversing gravity is.

● **Reverse gravity and stay fit** The unrelenting pull of gravity on your body year after year takes its toll, contributing to sagging muscles on the face and body, poor circulation in the legs and the kind of postural degeneration – humped shoulders and collapsed rib-cages – which can begin as early as the teens to make one look middle-aged. Reversing gravity for a few minutes each day can not only help prevent these age-related signs from developing, but can also help remove them once they have. You can practise inversion by using a slant board, by hanging from a rope which has been well secured from a door frame, or by using gravity boots for knee and back swings. But you shouldn't do the true yoga postures without the help of a good teacher or you can do more harm than good by compressing the vertebrae in the neck.

● **Lymph magic** Inverting your body for a few minutes each day encourages efficient lymphatic drainage, thereby improving the nourishment to and the elimination from the cells of muscles and skin. Over a few weeks, both the functions and the look of your skin improve, muscles are toned and cellulite diminishes.

● **Brain fuel** Hanging upside down increases the flow of fresh blood through your brain's cells, stimulating them. This acts as a kind of tonic to the mind – particularly in people who tire easily. One of the most useful attributes of hanging we personally find is its ability to combat mental staleness at the end of a long, hard day. Five minutes of flooding your brain with rich, oxygenated blood while you are stretched out in a position of complete relaxation is worth several hours of unwinding and leaves you refreshed and clear-headed.

● **Back therapy** *par excellence* Inversion can be great therapy for back problems as well. It offers a gravity-controlled means of traction which relieves pressure on protruding invertebral discs and compressed nerve roots. This, coupled with the stimulation it offers to circulation and lymphatic drainage and its usefulness in eliminating long-term areas of tension in the body, means that it can be enormously helpful in the treatment of low back pain. We know a great many previous back pain sufferers for whom it has been a godsend. They tend to become so enthusiastic about hanging that they think it is the ideal treatment for any back ailment whatsoever. It isn't. While it can be enormously helpful in many cases of even the most resistant back problems, there are others for which it does nothing and some for which it can actually be counter-productive. It is not good for acute lumbago, for instance, or for a few cases of sciatica. And it is certainly to be avoided by anyone with high or low blood pressure, a damaged or loose ankle joint or ligament, a hiatus hernia, an artificial hip or artificial lower limb joints. It is important to check with your doctor before using any kind of inversion equipment for therapeutic purposes. But for the well, the athlete, or the woman or man intent upon preserving youthful functioning and looks, it offers real help.

● **Make your own slant board** Take a board as long as your body and between 12 and 18 inches (30 to 45cm) wide. Place enough thick books or wooden blocks under one end to raise it 24 inches (61 cm) off the floor. Then lie down on it with your feet at the raised end. This is an excellent time to put on a sleeping mask or to place a piece of dark fabric over your eyes to block out light and do a meditation or visualization exercise. Fifteen minutes of this gentle form of inversion will refresh and revive you when you are fatigued. It will also bring a healthy, wonderful glow to your skin.

● **Scarafaggio** Our favourite inversion trick is lying on your back on the floor with your arms and legs drawn up, knees bent and just hanging there in the air – just like the Italian cockroach, from which its name comes, stranded on its back. The only problem is that it can be slightly embarrassing to be suddenly spotted doing it by someone who isn't privy to the special inside information about what it can do for you.

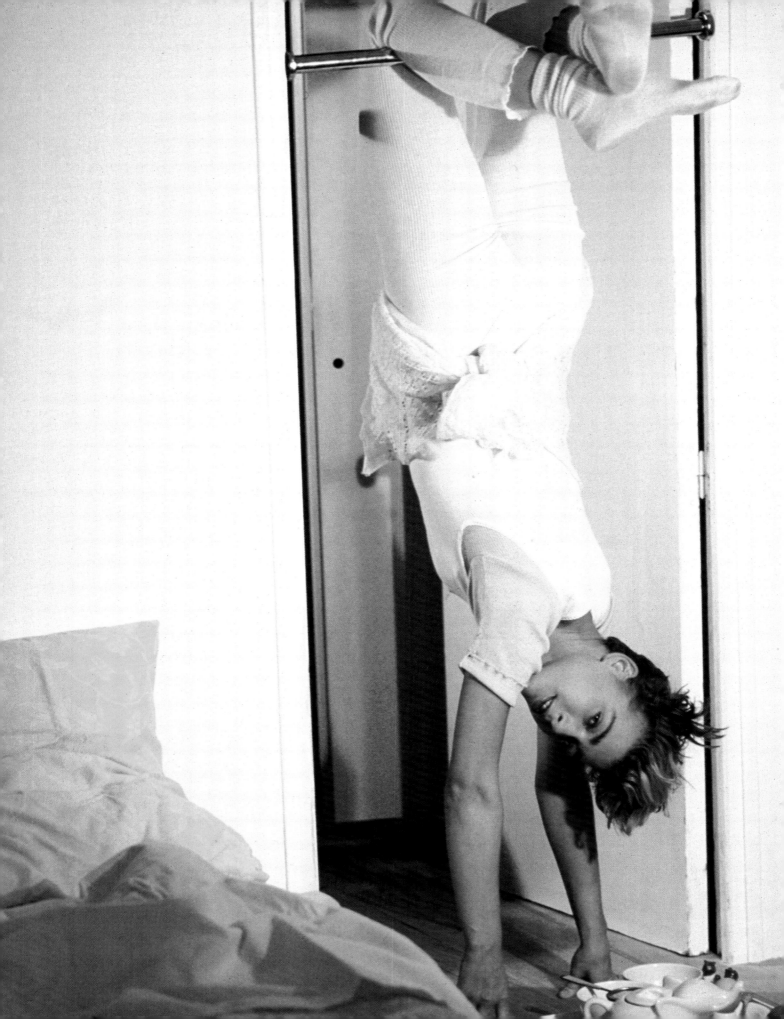

SUN WORSHIP

There would be no life without the sun. Hitting our biosphere, its rays give energy to plants who through photosynthesis turn it into carbohydrates, proteins and fats which make it possible for us and the animals we eat to exist. It is not these visible rays which appear to be the most important for health; it is the ultraviolet waves which are slightly shorter. They are the most biologically active of the whole spectrum. Unfortunately it is this UV light which is most easily blocked by clothes, sunglasses and windows.

In the late nineteenth century two scientists discovered that sunlight would destroy bacteria. Then in 1903 Niels Finsen won a Nobel prize for having successfully treated tuberculosis with UV light. Researchers found that exposing large areas of the body to UV light even once could dramatically lower high blood pressure, rebalance blood-sugar in diabetes, increase the number of lymphocytes in the blood, thereby strengthening the immune system, and decrease levels of cholesterol in the blood. So sunlight was much favoured for three generations as a way of treating illness and of helping well people stay well. Then, with the discovery of anti-bacterial drugs such as sulphanilamide and later penicillin in the early 1940s, suddenly respect for sun power waned. Doctors began to treat the notion that it could heal as nothing more than superstition based on the placebo effect. By the 1970s the great sun had fallen so much from favour that current medical opinion viewed it largely as a destructive power – the major culprit in skin aging and the cause of skin cancer. Now that opinion is beginning to shift. For there are many other factors such as the highly refined Western diet and pollution in our food, water and air which seem to be at fault. The sun is beginning to appear as little more than the trigger – a trigger which is only pulled if you get too much of it.

● **Sun fitness** One of the most interesting areas of research into the beneficial effects of sunlight shows that sunlight is an effective force in helping to keep your body fit. The ancient Romans always trained their gladiators in full sunlight in the belief that it strengthens and enlarges muscles. And indeed it does. Recent evidence shows that sunlight has a metabolic effect on the body which parallels physical training. Many of the beneficial effects of regular aerobic exercise can be had, to a somewhat lesser degree, by regular exposure to sunlight. The most exciting benefits to the body are when both sunlight and exercise are taken together. Studies show that this combination improves your resistance to illness, heightens mental functions and even makes you feel happier than either on its own.

● **Hormone trigger** Sunlight also has a powerful effect on the body's hormone production, first because it stimulates glands themselves and second because it causes hormone production by the skin itself. When UV light hits the skin it spurs the production of sex hormones. The oestrogen-like substance made in the skin is drawn into the bloodstream and has been shown experimentally to be powerful enough to trigger the menstrual cycle in neutered female mice and rats. Some doctors report remarkable success in treating women without menstrual periods through sunlight exposure. They have also used sunbathing as a cure for severe menopausal symptoms. UV radiation even seems to stimulate the thyroid gland, causing it to increase hormone production, heightening the basal metabolism and spurring the body to burn more calories. How then do you gain the sun's benefits without becoming one of its casualties?

● **Sensible sun worship** The answer is certainly not to run to your nearest sunbed salon for a dose of tan. The modern sunbed is anathema to most light researchers as it is to most dermatologists. Light researchers shun it because the kind of UV light it produces is greatly distorted – nothing like natural sunlight. It is highly unbalanced and may have long-term negative effects on the body. Dermatologists disapprove of modern sunbeds because people using them tend to get very high doses of UVA which is suspected of playing a major part in the early aging of skin. And what about sunlamps? They are definitely second best and should only be used when natural sunlight is not available. If you do buy a sunlamp it should never produce frequency below 290nm and it should give full UVA and UVB radiation.

The best way to get your daily dose of sunlight for the benefit of your health and good mood is to sunbathe outdoors for carefully controlled periods of time, and as naked as possible, since the greater the surface of the body which is exposed to UV light the better the results. This can be done even in winter if you are lucky enough to have an area sheltered from the wind on all sides. In the summer sunbathe only before 11 a.m. or after 3

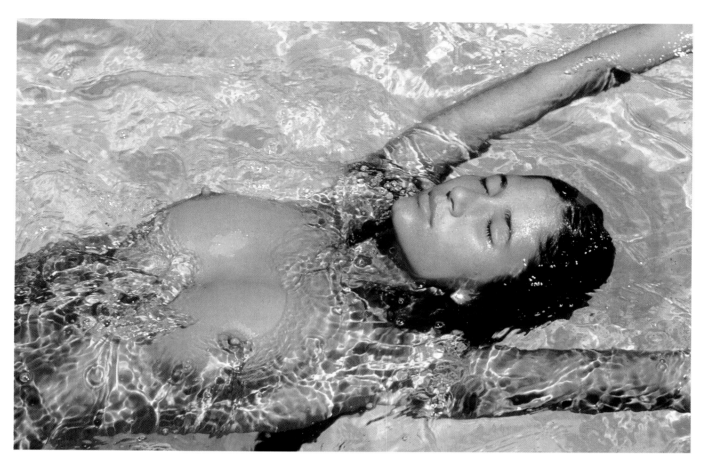

p.m. when the sun is not at its strongest. Start with as little as 2 minutes on each part of your body – front, back, sides – in full summer sun and then gradually lengthen your time in the sun by 1 minute on each area every day, working up to 10 or 15 minutes on each part. If a few hours after sunbathing you find your skin turning slightly pink, then don't lengthen your exposure again for several days. You should always keep to a level which does not allow you to burn or your sunbaths will be counter-productive.

Sunbathing for health should be done with clean, dry skin – *no lotions or oils.* Sunlight taken in this way in small doses will never dry the skin. Instead, thanks to the hormones it stimulates, it will tend to give your skin a lovely smoothness. However you go about it, one thing is sure: if you get regular exposure to sunlight, provided it is not in excessive quantities (beach bums take note!), you are likely to look and feel much better than ever before.

TAN LIGHTLY AND SAFELY
Everybody knows that sun damages skin. UV radiation is the single most powerful accelerator of skin aging to which you are likely to be exposed. It causes collagen to break down so that skin wrinkles, weakens elastin so that it sags, and brings about unsightly pigmentation blotches which are sure signs of growing old. Trouble is,

many women love a tan. Until recently you have had two choices – tan and age or stay pale and preserve your skin. Now that is changing, thanks to new advances in cosmetic chemistry and new formulations which make use of them. And while no woman in her right mind should toast herself in the sun, with a clear understanding of what is involved in the tanning process, you should be able to have your cake and eat it too.

Most of the highly sophisticated new suntanning products are aimed at optimizing this natural protective process while guarding against damage within the skin. They incorporate highly selective UVA and UVB filters which transmit only a controlled amount of UV radiation – just enough to stimulate the formation of melanin, which is responsible for the development of a tan. Many are also formulated to increase melanin synthesis in the melanosomes. This they can do by providing skin with substances such as the amino acid tyrosine which help accelerate the formation of melanin in the skin. Many of the new products are also designed to influence the formation of keratinocytes, which carry the pigments to the skin's surface, so that they have a good capacity for renewal and thus maintaining perfect integrity, and so that your skin is in the best possible state of hydration, elasticity, smoothness and firmness. The melanin-stimulating products are best used for several days *before* heading out into the sun.

Body Time

103

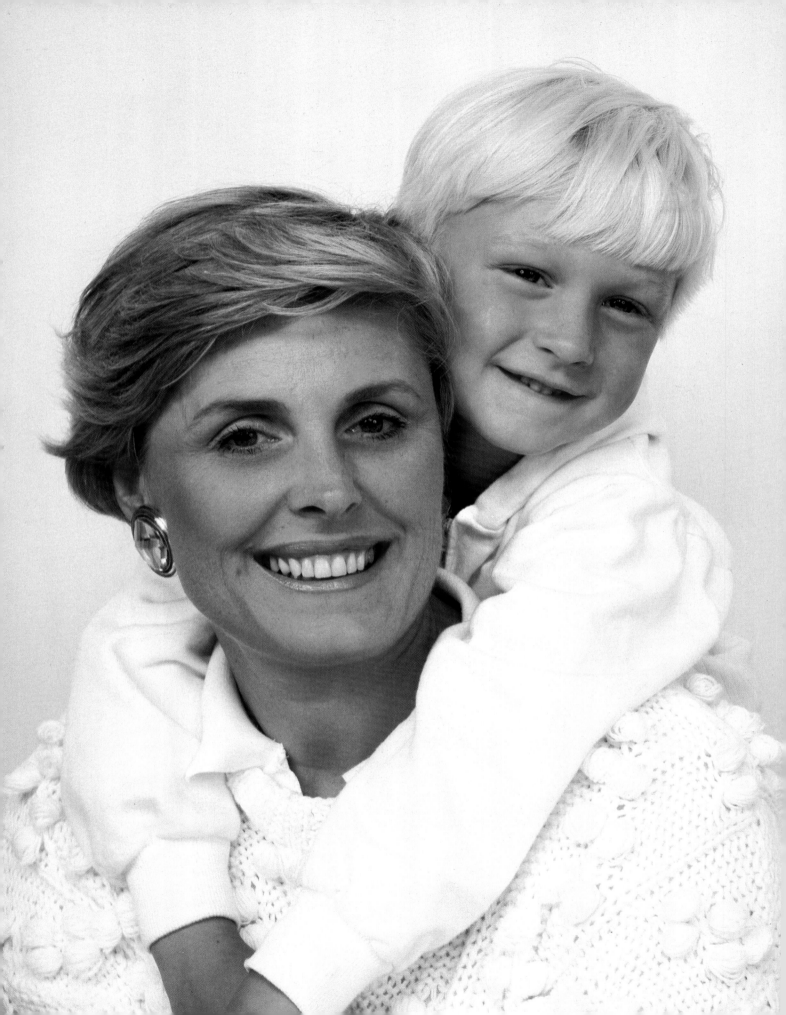

BEAT TIME

Time passing can be a worry. Most women look in the mirror around 30 and start to fret over fine lines around their eyes or thinning hair or stiffening joints. Take heart if you are one of these. While getting older is a fact of life for all of us to cope with, there are nonetheless numerous safe things you can do to slow down the process and protect yourself from the ravages of premature aging, whether it begins to show itself in sagging skin and wrinkles or the development of degenerative illnesses such as arthritis, cancer or coronary heart disease. Getting older is inevitable; the degeneration which often accompanies it, for most of us, is *not*.

There are many theories about aging – why it occurs, how it takes place and what can be done to retard it. At one time they seemed contradictory. Now most of them appear to link up with a kind of pattern which can help guide us in slowing down the process. Each plays its part in the understanding of what we call aging. Taken together, these theories provide us with good guidelines about what we should and shouldn't do to protect ourselves against the ravages of time. Learn about them and put them into practice *now* – whether you are 20 or 70. Using them is like putting money in the bank. They will create energy and good looks on which you can draw for years to come.

Keep slim Statistics show that the number of years of life lost from being overweight are from 4 to 11, not to mention the enormous waste of energy and the lowered vitality that comes from carrying excess baggage. *Now* is the time to shed it.

Don't smoke The years lost if you are a smoker vary from about 4, if you smoke, say, 10 cigarettes a day, to nearly 20 years for women who smoke 40 or more.

Eat well but not too much Scientists estimate that the lifespan increase which can be brought about from living on a good diet of whole foods which is low in fat, moderate in protein and high in fresh fruits and vegetables is somewhere between 10 and 20 years. The benefits, from increased energy to heightened well-being, that accrue by following such a way of eating are measureless. Nutritional supplements can help too.

Do a periodic internal spring-clean Detoxifying your body two or three times a year with an apple fast of a few days or spending a week or two on raw foods is an absolute must unless you happen to live like a nun, exercise like a top athlete and eat like a yogi. The detoxification 'cure' (see pp. 120–1) helps eliminate wastes from tissues and breaks negative habit patterns which are associated with rapid aging. It also gives you a chance to take a new look at yourself and your life – essential if you are not to crystallize into mechanical ways of thinking and being.

Get moving The loss of years due to lack of exercise is estimated to be between 6 and 9. Exercise is vital for preserving your skin quality and look, for protecting arteries from furring up and for keeping your immune system functioning at peak. Time to get moving!

YOUTH FOODS

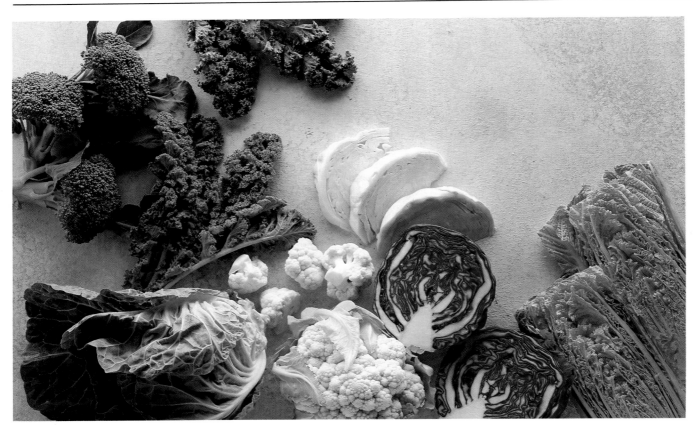

How and what you eat has a lot to do with how rapidly your body ages. The average Western diet, which is high in calories, high in fats, and contains far more protein than the body needs for optimum health, is about the worst you can follow if you want to slow the rate at which you age. So think twice before you tuck into that huge steak.

Most of us eat more than we need. Every extra calorie you consume above the absolute minimum your body needs you can count as a mark against you and a mark for Father Time. But this doesn't mean going on some kind of slimming regime permanently. For *low calorie* is only the first half of the diet equation for preventing premature aging. The other half is equally important: *high potency*. Just what does this mean? It means that you have to make every calorie count, not just in terms of energy, but also in terms of maintaining a high level of essential nutrients (vitamins, minerals and essential fatty acids) as well as fibre which your body needs to function in peak condition. Roy Walford, an American age researcher famous for his well-substantiated findings, put it this way: 'You need *under nutrition* without *malnutrition*.' So instead of eating, say, 2500–3000 calories a day, as most people now do, you need to cut your calorie intake to about 1800.

● **Beware of excess proteins** Women's magazines are traditional advocates of the 'high protein diet'. They are full of articles urging you to eat lots of protein if you want to have strong healthy hair and nails. But they are mistaken. Most of us eat far more protein than we need, with the consequence that we not only tend to age more rapidly, but also that we lose minerals from our bones. That is why a sensible diet for longevity and age retardation takes no more than 20 per cent of its calories from proteins.

● **An anti-aging food style** For a high-energy life style which helps keep you young and and vigorous while others are falling by the wayside, this what to go for and what to steer clear of:

YOUTH-MAKERS	YOUTH-BREAKERS
wholegrain cereals	highly processed foods
wholegrain breads	refined cereals
pulses	white bread and
fresh vegetables	anything made from
fresh fruit	white flour
fish, game and free-range poulty in moderation	sugar and sweets
	artificially coloured and flavoured foods
liver from organically raised animals	tinned meats and fish
	smoked meats and fish

HIGH-POWERED FOODS

But there is even more to it than this. In order to ensure that you are getting the highest possible complement of vitamins and minerals, you should also see that you eat at least half of your foods raw. And there are a few high-powered foods which have something special to offer for health and youth. Try to make a place for them in the other half.

● **Liver** Liver is packed with B-complex vitamins, anti-stress minerals, protein (and a little fat), trace elements and minerals such as potassium, sodium and magnesium. Liver from organically raised animals is also a safe source of the sulphur amino acids, which are excellent free radical scavengers that help protect from oxidation damage (see p. 108). And liver is one of the richest natural sources for vitamin A, another anti-oxidant nutrient which is essential for skin health and involved in all the body's repair and growth processes.

● **Eggs** Eggs have been much maligned in recent years because of their cholesterol content, which was once assumed to raise cholesterol levels in the blood significantly and therefore believed to contribute to coronary heart disease. Recent thinking on the subject is changing however. For the egg yolk is a balanced combination of essential nutrients, offering not only cholesterol, but also zinc, sulphur, iron and lecithin, all of which enable your body to convert the cholesterol into valuable steroid hormones which help to protect *against* disease and aging. Eating several eggs a week can do a lot of good. They are low in fat, rich in top-quality protein and vitamin A, as well as many of the B-complex vitamins. They have a high content of the sulphur amino acids methionine and cysteine, as well as selenium – all important anti-aging substances.

● **Sunflower seeds** Higher in protein than any other seed (and even than many cuts of meat), sunflower seeds are a concentrated source of nutritional protection. They are a rich source of vitamin E (one of the vitamins difficult to get in good amounts in the average Western diet) plus unsaturated fatty acids and many of the B-complex vitamins, particularly B6, which women on the Pill need in greater quantities than normal. Sunflower seeds are also high in important minerals such as iron, potassium, iodine and magnesium.

● **Blackstrap molasses** A tablespoonful of blackstrap molasses supplies as much calcium as a glass of milk and as much iron as nine eggs. It is an extraordinarily valuable food for women who tend to suffer from anaemia. Blackstrap molasses boasts large quantities of the B-complex vitamins and more potassium than any other food. It is also rich in magnesium, phosphorus, copper and vitamin E, and is a great natural sweetener for yoghurt or drinks.

● **Seaweed** Sea plants have a natural advantage over land plants because they grow in mineral-rich sea water. Seaweed, or kelp, contains all the necessary minerals in a beautifully balanced and easily assimilable form. Kelp is an excellent source of iodine which helps protect against the destructive power of radioactivity in the atmosphere and strengthens nails and hair. It is also rich in B-complex vitamins, vitamins D, E and K, calcium and magnesium. You can use it dried as a salt substitute or take tablets of it.

● **Garlic** Garlic is a powerful detoxifier which is a must in every woman's diet. This evil-smelling little bulb has two important parts to play in the prevention of aging. First, it has the ability to clear out wastes from your body and render harmless toxic substances which cause cell damage. Second, it can lower serum-cholesterol which helps protect against atherosclerosis, one of the dangerous manifestations of age degeneration. If you are offended by the taste of garlic you can swallow tiny capsules of garlic oil bought from health food stores. They leave no after-taste and do not affect your breath. In any case, garlic breath can be eliminated by chewing fresh parsley.

● **Cabbage and raw green vegetables** Cabbage is a rich source of important anti-aging sulphur compounds. Like most leafy green vegetables, it also contains good quantities of vitamins and minerals (providing of course it has been grown in healthy soils and is eaten fresh). All raw vegetables are a good source of dietary fibre which has been shown to be important in protecting the body from the harmful effects of radiation. Many are also diuretic and so help the body process liquid waste.

● **Wheatgerm** The heart of the wheat, wheatgerm, is the richest known source of vitamin E. It also has good amounts of the B-complex vitamins and iron. And it is a superb source of protein which can be sprinkled on salads and wholegrain cereals. Because wheatgerm oxidizes rapidly due to its oil content, it should be kept in an airtight container and refrigerated.

TO AGE OR NOT TO AGE

The aging of skin, like the aging of your entire body, is a multi-dimensional process which involves many mechanisms, both at a cellular level and in your body as a whole. And while nobody has any pat answers about how to stop it completely, most age researchers agree that the changes which occur to skin – from its loss of elasticity and firmness to wrinkling itself – take place as a result of damage done on a molecular level to the cells themselves and to the collagen surrounding them. The culprits which cause most of this damage are some highly reactive molecules called *free radicals*.

RAPISTS AND WRINKLES

Free radicals are species of atoms or molecules which are dangerous simply because they are electromagnetically unbalanced. This causes them to react with other molecules causing damage. They can disrupt the genetic material in the cells all over your body so that it no longer reproduces accurately. They can damage precious cell membranes through which nourishment and oxygen must pass and can also cause proteins in the cells and collagen itself to cross-link. Recently, free radical damage has been linked to the development of many diseases, from cancer and coronary heart disease to arthritis and environmental allergies. Prevent free radical damage and you should go a long way towards slowing down the rate at which you age.

Gerentologist Alex Comfort once likened a free radical to 'a convention delegate away from his wife: it's a highly reactive chemical agent that will combine with anything that's around.' Other researchers believe that free radicals can be better compared to rapists whose union with other molecules, willing or unwilling, is nothing less than clear attack. Free radicals can cut other molecules down the middle, chop pieces out of them, distort cellular information and generally wreak havoc with living systems. They can cause cell injury, inflammation and destruction to parts of cells, cell walls, collagen fibres (the body's most important structural protein) and many other things.

When free radicals react with molecules of protein in the cell or in the tissue these long-chained proteins become *cross-linked*, which means that they get molecularly bound together and tangled. As a result, your tissues lose their suppleness, skin wrinkles, veins and arteries become hardened and more inclined to build up

deposits of cholesterol and even your chances of developing a cancerous growth increase. The genetic material in your cells (which is necessary for cell division and tissue repair) also becomes garbled. It is because of the damage caused by free radicals that you are warned to protect your skin from sunlight, avoid cigarette smoke and drink little alcohol.

● **Cosmetic damage** The damage that free radicals can do to the elastin and collagen in your skin's connective tissue is particularly worrying from a cosmetic point of view. It makes your skin sag and causes your muscles to lose their firmness. Collagen, which is often considered the mortar of the skin's cells, makes up some 25 per cent of your body's protein. It lends structural support to all living cells. When collagen and other connective proteins are young they have an almost gel-like quality. For your cells to be nourished, nutrients have to pass through the collagen network. Through this network, too, are eliminated the cell's waste products. Collagen which has become cross-linked as a result of free radical attack is no longer gel-like. It tends to impede proper cell nutrition and waste elimination and therefore lowers cell vitality and eventually the vitality of the whole organism. An important source of free radical harm in relation to aging comes from exposing your skin unprotected to the sun. Free radical damage and oxidation can also result from even low levels of radiation, such as the type emitted by microcomputers or word processors. Stay away from environmental pollution, too, if you want to protect yourself from early aging. For, different as these things are, all of them can trigger free radical production in the cells through a process called peroxidation.

ANTI-OXIDANT DEFENCES

Your body in its wisdom has devised a number of mechanisms to protect itself from free radical damage. But our twentieth-century environment is too full of external sources of free radicals. They include radiation of all sorts, from the sun's ultraviolet rays to emanations from nuclear power stations and even the electromagnetic fields set up by high-tension electrical installations. They also include air pollutants such as ozone, nitrogen dioxide, sulphur dioxide, cigarette smoke, solvents, pesticides and drugs; polyvalent metals such as lead, cadmium and aluminium; certain preservatives such as sodium nitrite which is used for bacon and luncheon meats; as well as certain foods, particularly those lacking in freshness. The eating of too much food, and the toxic residues from illness or prolonged emotional stress as well, can also spur free radical reactions and cross-linkage.

Even the oxygen we breathe, which is so essential to all life's processes, is an important factor in bringing about free radical damage, not only because the majority of free radical reactions involve oxygen, but because oxygen in certain forms can actually behave like a free radical itself. Since the 1950s gerentologists have reported success in retarding aging and promoting longevity using chemical substances – both natural and artificial – which protect living systems from oxidation or free radical damage. Free radical scavengers include substances such as zinc, vitamin C, vitamin E, vitamin A and selenium.

These substances which protect against peroxidation and deactivate free radicals are usually grouped together under the label 'anti-oxidants'. Many age experts now agree that anti-oxidants can create a bastion of defence against degeneration not only in the skin but also in the body as a whole. Anti-oxidants can slow down destructive peroxidation of lipids or fats in your body. They also react harmlessly with free radicals, deactivating them before they can do harm to cell membranes, genetic material and other proteins.

Anti-oxidants come in two varieties: natural and artificial. The natural anti-oxidants are simple nutritional elements which occur naturally in the foods we eat. These include ascorbic acid, vitamins A, E and many of the B-complex, zinc, selenium and some free amino acids. They are increasingly considered a vital part of any serious programme for ageless aging. The artificial ones, such as the food preservatives BHA and BHT, are best left alone.

MEET THE YOUTH GUARDIANS

These nutritional substances have each been shown in animal studies to be effective tools in the prevention of premature aging. Aging experts agree that most of us age prematurely. We come nowhere near our potential for longevity, vitality and lasting good looks. Anti-oxidants help prevent oxidation damage and cross-linking and may even aid in the correction of damage already

sustained. They also help strengthen the functioning of the immune system.

That is why we call them the youth guardians: zinc, selenium, vitamin C, vitamin A, vitamin E, pantothenic acid, vitamins B1 and B6, as well as the sulphur amino acids, methionine and cysteine. If they are taken as supplements, they should always be taken in a balanced formula which includes all the other minerals and vitamins which are needed for them to work biochemically within your body. Make friends with the youth guardians and they will serve you well.

ANTI-AGING FORMULA

THE VITAMINS

Vitamin A	15,000–25,000 IU
Beta-carotene	15–45 mg
Vitamin C	5–10 g
Bioflavonoids	250–2000 mg
Vitamin E	400–800 IU
Vitamin D	400 IU
Vitamin B1	100–1000 mg
Vitamin B2	100–300 mg
Vitamin B3	250–3000 mg
Vitamin B5	250–3000 mg
Vitamin B6	50–150 mg
Vitamin B12	100–500 mcg with sorbitol
Vitamin B15	150–250 mg
Folic acid	800–5000 mcg
PABA	250–750 mg
Biotin	150–750 mg
Choline	500–2000 mg
Inositol	500–3000 mg

THE MINERALS

Calcium	1000–2000 mg
Magnesium	500–1000 mg
Zinc	10–25 mg
Manganese	10–25 mg
Molybedenum	250–1000 mcg
Chromium	20–200 mcg
or GFT form if possible	100–400 mcg
Selenium	100–300 mcg

AMINO ACIDS

L-methionine	500–1500 mg
L-cysteine	500–1500 mg

YOUTH SUPPLEMENTS

As your body ages, many essential hormones are in increasingly short supply, while at the same time imbalances between various hormones and the glands that secrete them tend to develop. Glands, or more specifically endocrine glands, secrete hormones directly into your bloodstream. In the body there are complex biochemical cycles involving hormones moving from one gland to trigger actions in organs and other glands. There are also superbly controlled feedback loops for slowing or stopping the functions of another gland or organ when a particular task is finished.

RAW GLANDULARS

According to experts in cell therapy – the European anti-aging method of injecting fresh cells from animals into the human body – one of the reasons why it can be useful in restoring vitality to an aging organism and improving immunity is because the majority of cells used are taken from endocrine glands, which can help to restore depleted hormones near to normal. For many years the idea of giving raw whole-glandular therapy was dismissed, but now there is evidence that substances in properly prepared glandular tissues – such as enzymes, hormones, polypeptides, essential fatty acids and even prostaglandins – can have clinically significant effects which may account for their therapeutic value in oral glandular therapy.

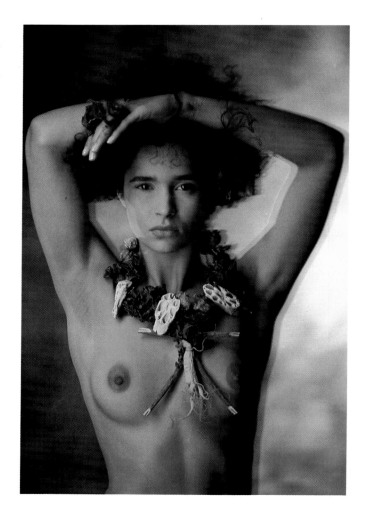

There are a number of glands which are available for oral use. They can be purchased from health food shops and by post from manufacturers of nutritional supplements. The best glandulars are freeze-dried. It is very important to make sure that the glandular materials themselves come, not from animals which have been raised on feed lots, but from livestock which has been grazed in open fields, and that the supplement has been prepared in such a way that each tablet is protected from stomach acid.

The most commonly used gland is the thymus because this gland, which is often called 'the master gland of immunity', governs immune functions which in turn play such central roles in how rapidly the body ages. Other common endocrine glands used in anti-aging treatment include the pituitary, the pancreas, the adrenals and the male and female sex glands. Raw glandulars are usually taken for a period of about six weeks at a time a couple of times a year. They are best taken up when your body has good supplies of the nutrients needed to make use of them – vitamins C, A, E, folic acid, B6, zinc, B12, manganese, B1 and B2. Most glandulars are given in amounts of 200–1000 mg a day in two doses.

Multiple whole glandulars are usually a combination of tissues, such as liver, brain, stomach and heart, together with pancreas, thyroid, thymus, adrenal, pituitary and pineal glands. They often come together with a whole ovarian and uterus tissue for women and a prostate and orchic (taken from the testicles) for men. The multiple glandulars are often considered an excellent overall twice-yearly treatment to boost the body's functions as a whole.

Youth Herbs

Throughout history certain plants have been credited with an ability to prolong youth and restore vitality which has been lost as years pass. Thanks to recent research, much of which has been carried out by top scientists in the Soviet Union, we know that many of the old-fashioned youth herbs *do* work and in very specific ways. Substances such as ginseng and eleuthrococcus (which is often called Siberian ginseng) have what are called *adaptogenic* properties. Taken regularly over several weeks, they are able to enhance your body's resistance to illness, aging, fatigue and stress. In short, they help strengthen and rebalance your whole system.

● **Eleuthrococcus or Siberian ginseng** A prickly plant known as 'devil's shrub', Siberian ginseng has beautiful yellow and purple flowers, but it is the hot and spicy roots which hold its health-enhancing properties. It has been shown in scientific experiments to strengthen resistance to illness, fatigue and degeneration. It is also a mild stimulant and therefore should never be taken at bedtime. People who have used it report better sleep patterns, increased stamina, improved memory and enhanced athletic performance. Eleuthrococcus is also a natural anti-oxidant. It helps protect your body against the kind of free radical damage which results in the cross-linking of proteins and leads to wrinkling and sagging skin (see p.108). It even appears to have anti-cancer properties.

● **Ginseng** Another 'medicine for the well', ginseng has been widely investigated and found to have properties similar to eleuthrococcus. It is often used to eliminate toxicity in the body because of its anti-oxidant properties and it is a classical antidote to fatigue, weakness and anaemia. It is a super tool for staving off exhaustion and helps lower blood pressure which is too high, heightens men's sexual facilities and is a gentle stimulant to the central nervous system. Ginseng is also considered a good antidote to depression, but it is a better anti-aging tool for men and women past the menopause than it is for pre-menopausal women. Be sure to get a good source of the herb, either on its own or in a tonic. Many ginseng products are worthless because they have been unwisely processed.

● **Sarsaparilla and damiana** While the rest of us rave about the potential of hormone replacement therapy or dispute its safety, in Mexico herbal doctors insist that they have been doing virtually the same thing for years with special 'rejuvenating herbs' which, they claim, have none of the side-effects of drugs. These herbs are used for restoring a youthful appearance and for retaining the proper functioning of the endocrine system. Two of the most important are damiana (*Turnera aphrodisiaca*), a small shrub whose leaves are dried and used as tea, and sarsaparilla (*Smilax medica* or *S. regalii*), a tropical plant grown in Honduras, Mexico, Jamaica and Ecuador as well as China and Japan.

Damiana has for generations been used as an aphrodisiac and a remedy for sexual impotence, but according to the directors of the two most exclusive health spas in Mexico, it is also an excellent nerve tonic and a natural diuretic. Sarsaparilla is supposed to be a potent blood purifier and powerful antidote to any kind of poisoning. Most important of all, researchers have shown that the plant is a surprisingly rich source of testosterone- and progesterone-like (male and female sex hormones), as well as the adrenal-like, hormones.

Gerentologists point out that one of the most important causes of aging (both in appearance and general well-being) is the slowing down of hormone production in the endocrine and sex glands. Sarsaparilla supplies some of those missing hormones.

Damiana is prepared like any other herb tea: one teaspoon of the dried leaves to one cup of boiling water, steeped for five minutes. It is served twice daily in many Mexican health spas. Sarsaparilla roots are boiled in spring water (1 oz [25 g] of root to each 20 fl oz [2½ cups/1 litre] water) for 25 minutes. This concoction is drunk hot both morning and evening. Both damiana and sarsaparilla are available in shops specializing in herbs.

If you are going to take any of these plant substances, be sure that you are buying top-quality plants or products. For when many plant substances, such as eleuthrococcus, are heated too much or over-processed, their anti-aging, anti-stress properties are greatly reduced. Youth herbs are best used as a 'cure' in the French sense – that is, two or three times a year for a period of from two to six weeks. Most need to be taken on an empty stomach and all of them must be taken every day to work their natural wonders. Herbal products are very different from the drugs most people are used to. They work slowly but steadily at altering your biochemistry from the inside and they must be allowed time to change things for the better.

Beat Time

COSMETIC AID

Once cosmetics offered little more than beautiful jars and empty promises to women hoping for help against age-related damage to their skin. No longer. Thanks to recent advances in cosmetic chemistry and in-depth studies of the processes involved in skin aging, there is much which can be done cosmetically to alter the functions of aging skin so that it looks and behaves like young skin. And the most expensive skin care products are by no means necessarily the best. There are a number of middle-price treatment products which are excellent. In addition to the two skin essentials – a moisturizer (preferably based on essential fatty acids) and a sunscreen which you wear summer and winter with or without make-up – as well as daily care (see pp. 58–9), there are a number of other anti-aging skin care products which can do useful things to help protect from aging and to renew and regenerate aged skin.

ANTI-AGING SKIN CARE

● **Stimulating DNA repair** Several products now available are designed to stimulate the repair of genetic material in your skin cells which has been damaged by ultraviolet radiation and free radicals (see p. 108). They come in various forms – creams, lotions and drops – which you spread on skin after cleansing in the evening, since the night-time is when your cells' own repair mechanisms are at their most active.

● **Heightening oxygenation of cells** As skin ages, the rate at which your cells use oxygen tends to decline and with it the skin's metabolic functions. Many of the anti-aging creams and ampoules are specifically designed to enhance oxygen use by skin cells and to stimulate the cells of older skin to behave more like younger ones.

● **Increasing cell turnover** Another slow-down which occurs with age is the rate at which your skin cells reproduce from the basal layer between the dermis (the true skin) and the epidermis (the outer surface of the skin that we see). Some anti-aging cosmetics are designed to heighten cell turnover either by biochemical stimulation or simply through exfoliation, where dead cells on the skin's surface are sloughed off mechanically via grainy scrubs. This both stimulates cell turnover and smooths out the surface of your skin, making it look polished, fresh and young.

● **Improving firmness** Thanks to the biochemical actions of various substances on the connective tissue

and the gel-like medium in which it sits, cosmetic science can also offer products which contain active ingredients that improve skin firmness.

● **A magic for skin** Vitamin A is not only one of the most potent of all the anti-oxidants you will find anywhere, it is also an excellent antidote to the dryness of skin which increases as you get older. There are few cosmetic products on the market yet which take advantage of the wonderful support which this nutrient can give skin. But, if you can stand the smell of fish oil on your face for 10–20 minutes a day (that's all it takes), this is a wonderful treatment to carry out after cleansing at night and before applying your night cream.

Take a capsule of pure vitamin A (it can be between 5000 and 25,000 IU). Pierce it with a pin and spread it upon your skin. Leave for 20–23 minutes and then tissue off or remove with the help of a non-alcoholic toner. Finally apply your ordinary night cream.

HOW OLD IS YOUR SKIN?

This simple test is an excellent way to find out just how much free radical damage and cross-linking has taken place in your skin. Place the palm of one hand flat against a table in front of you. Then, with the thumb and forefinger of the other hand, grasp a piece of the flesh on the back of the flattened hand and pull it up in a pinch, holding it there for a second or two. Now let go and notice how quickly it returns to its original place – so that every ridge and trace of the pinch disappears. On a very young hand where little oxidation damage and cross-linking has occurred, skin will spring back in as little as an eighth of a second. With skin from an old body – say, over 70 or 80 – it can take several seconds.

PROTECTION RACKET

The single most aging force to which most of us are ever exposed is sunlight (see p. 102). This wonderful stuff which makes you feel so good when you are out in it and which brings the beautiful glowing tan can be a destroyer of skin. If you value your skin – particularly the skin of your face – and want to keep it smooth and glowing as the years pass, then protect it, not just when you are on the tennis court or the beach, but all day, every day of your life. This is not as difficult to do as you might imagine, for many of the best moisturizers contain effective sunscreens.

Beat Time

Wrinkle Release

The ideal way to deal with wrinkles is to prevent them by steering clear of sunlight and sunbeds, ensuring your diet is sparse but good, getting lots of aerobic exercise and using the specific anti-oxidant nutrients which help prevent free radical or oxidation damage and cross-linking. But you need to preserve your facial muscles in tone as well.

This can be done by sitting in front of a mirror and working your face muscles against the resistance offered by pressing your fingers into your face at specific areas. How face exercises are done is very important if you are going to do good and not harm. Never grimace or work your face without some kind of firm resistance, as it is this which encourages muscles to become larger, smoothing out hollows.

Neck Help
Let your head fall back as far as it will. Now bring your bottom lip over the top one. You will feel the large muscle which runs from the chin down the front of the neck (the platysma) tighten. Begin to open and close your mouth slowly and in rhythm. You can utter 'umumumum' if you like as you do so to create the rhythm. Now tilt your head to the right and repeat the same movement, then go to the left and repeat it again. Spend 1 minute doing the exercise in each of the three directions.

Single Chin
Again, put your head back, but this time place the knuckles of one hand just under your chin in the soft part behind the bone. Now, pressing firmly but gently, rock your head back and forth against the resistance of your hand for 1 minute.

No Crow's Feet
Two things cause crow's feet. One is squinting and the second is the way in which, without exercise, the muscles around your eyes (the orbicularis occuli) tend to become flaccid so they are unable to support the skin firmly. This exercise works those muscles, enlarging and toning them so that hollows under the eyes tend to be filled in and crow's-feet areas are plumped up and smoothed out. Place your fingertips over the crow's-feet area on both sides, now press firmly. Then try to wink first one eye and then the other. This should be impossible to do completely if you are exercising correctly. You will feel the muscles around your eyes tighten and relax in a rhythmic way. Even 1 minute of this each day will make your eyes look better very quickly.

Banish the Frown
Frown lines are nasty and impossible to get rid of unless you break yourself of the habit of frowning which has caused them, as well as following this exercise routine for 1–2 minutes each

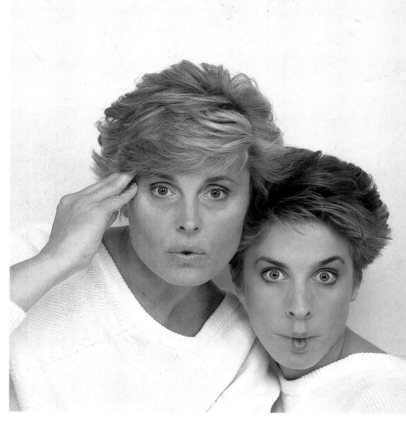

day. Place the fingertips of both hands along the upper brow and press firmly. Now try to frown and then release the frown rhythmically. If you are doing it right no crease will form between your brows.

Circulation Booster
Finish off by helping to nourish and relax the facial tissue you have been working by placing both hands first at the sides of your forehead and then across it, at the tops of the cheekbones, at the sides of the nose, under the cheeks, at the sides of the jaw and on the chin below the sides of your mouth one after the other. At each place, using the balls of your fingers, apply firm yet gentle pressure directly onto your face tissue and manipulate it gently by moving it in tiny circles beneath the skin. Your fingers must never pull against the skin itself. They stay in the same place. It is the tissue beneath the skin's surface which moves. Work the flesh for 5–10 seconds at each point. This will leave your skin glowing and your muscles feeling firm.

REJUVENATING MAKE-UP

Is there such a thing as rejuvenating make-up? Indeed there is. The right colours, skilfully applied, can make any face over 30 years old look younger. But make-up for the mature face should never be merely a means of adornment or decoration. It should be a way of strengthening what you already have – or making absolutely the best of everything.

One thing you will need is the proper tools to do good make-up: a sponge (either rubber or natural, for applying foundation or liquid blusher), a wedge-shaped brush (for colouring brows if they need it), an eyelash curler, two or three brushes (for loose powder, blending eye-shadow and applying pressed powder, blusher and highlighter), a good under-foundation make-up base or moisturizer (any make-up is only as good as the foundation it's applied on), two eyebrow brushes – old mascara brushes (clean) or small toothbrushes are ideal (one is for the brows, the other to feather your lashes after applying mascara) – and a sharpener for pencils.

Use concealer first: a cream, a stick, or one of the new pencil concealers in a shade just a little lighter than your own skin. Apply it generously with a clean brush, then press gently into the skin with your fingertip (since it is warm) and blend again with your brush into the surrounding area.

READY FOR FOUNDATION

Foundation is important after 35, since your skin tends to become unevenly textured as it ages. Light but effective coverage will smooth over all this. Choose a water-based one if your skin is oily, otherwise a liquid or cream emulsion is best. Match the colour to your jawline or neck so that you are all one shade when you finish. Always apply with a sponge from your chin upwards, blending and blending for a perfect finish, and set your foundation by gently blotting with a tissue placed open over the entire face.

DON'T LET EYE MAKE-UP SCARE YOU

It only looks bad when it's badly applied. And it can do much to bring youth to a face. Brows first. Most need nothing more than a little brushing – first against the direction in which they grow, then once or twice gently with it. If yours are really very thick, thin them by plucking individual hairs from *beneath* the brow, brushing them constantly up and down as you go to get a

clear view of your brow's natural line. If they are sparse, delicately fill them in by using a matt taupe or smoky eye-shadow or an eyebrow powder in a shade a bit lighter than your own. Finish off by giving your brows a good brushing to soften the lines.

● **Eye-liner is a must** Try it and see. To make a face more youthful, use it in two ways. First, draw a subtly coloured line to give just a hint of defining shadow at the outside corner of the lower lid and from about the middle of the upper lid outwards until the two lines meet. Use two different colours, say, a gentle lilac or grey or taupe for the underneath and deeper lilac, grey-blue or neutral brown for the upper line. Apply these lines finely, close to the roots of the lashes. Then, using a small brush or the tip of your finger, blend the colour towards the inner corner to soften it.

The second use of eye-liner is fabulous for rejuvenating the look of the eye. Take a flesh-coloured pencil and line the inside rim of the lower lids. This defines the eyes, opens them up and makes them sparkle. You can substitute a vivid blue or violet or bright green inside the lower lid for evening. This is the only place on a mature face that you should apply a strong line.

● **Eye-shadows for older lids** Never apply frosted or glittery colour to a crêpey eyelid or to any area of the face where there are fine lines. It only exaggerates them and is very aging indeed. Go instead for blushers and eye-shadows that are matt finish or have the *tiniest* hint of frost to them. The best eye-shadows for older lids are matt-pressed powders and very fine creams or gels. Apply them with fingers if you must, but use a soft eye-shadow brush to blend for a perfect finish.

● **Lashes need mascara** And lots of it. First curl them with an eyelash curler so the shadows they cast will be over your lids rather than over the eyes: they will look wider, brighter and younger. Apply mascara first on the tops of the upper lashes, then from below upwards, for a thicker look. And don't forget the lower ones. The best colours are brown or dark grey unless your lashes are very dark, in which case use black. Bright purples and blues don't work on mature faces.

BLUSHER

Creams and liquid blushers are the most natural, and are good on skin which tends to be dry. Apply them in dots from the top of the cheekbone and sweep them up

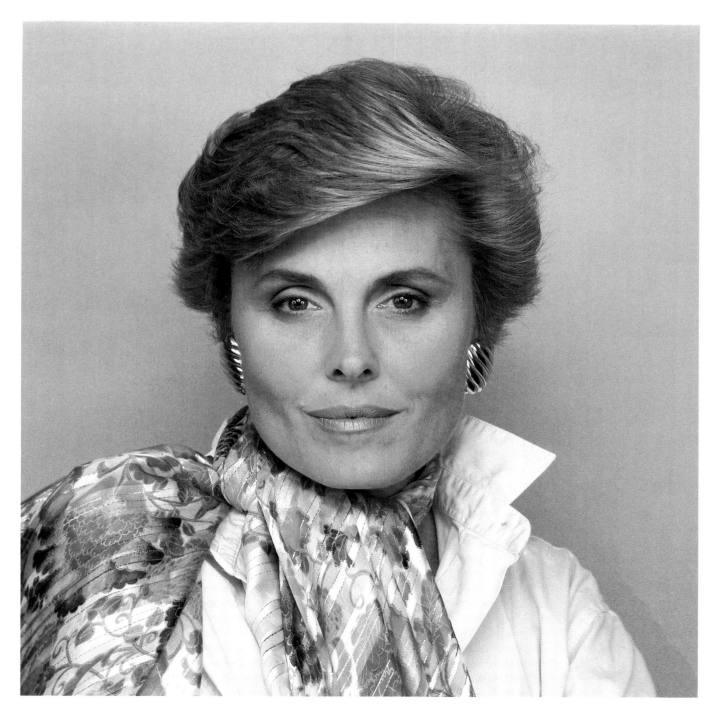

towards the temples as close to the eye as you can get. Put a drop on the bridge of your nose too, and a couple just under the hairline on your forehead; then blend with your sponge. Never apply colour anywhere beneath your cheekbones.

POWDER

Yes, by all means. It makes your skin texture look even, and 'sets' your make-up. Make sure it is very fine, without any sparkle, and completely colourless. Fluff it on loosely with a brush, then brush off any excess. The final trick for a dewy finish that lasts and lasts is this: close your eyes and spray the lot with a fine Evian mist. Then, separating two leaves of tissue from each other, lay one over your face to absorb the excess.

LIPS

If you have trouble with lipstick 'leaking' into the cracks around your lips, cover the outer edges of your upper lip with your foundation, blot it and apply powder before you apply pencil, gloss or lipstick. It gives a barrier that prevents lipstick from bleeding onto the skin.

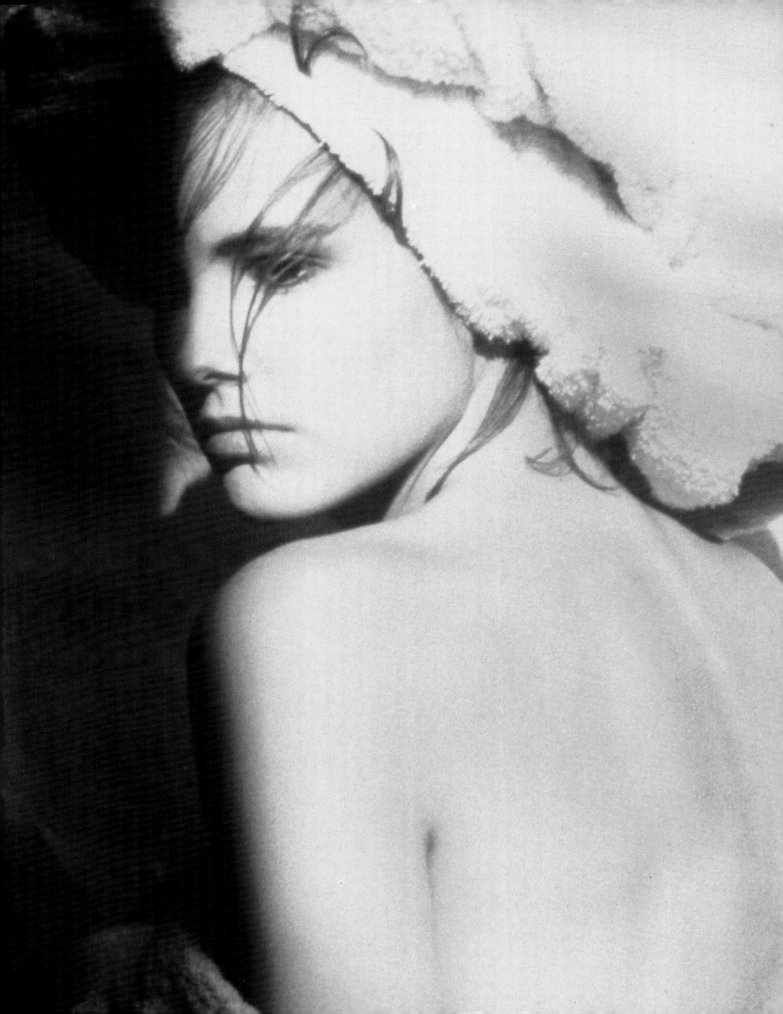

HELP TIME

Things don't always run smoothly – even for the most health-conscious of people. That is why simple, natural methods of problem-solving are such an essential part of a high-energy way of living. When something goes wrong – you get a cold or are struggling with chronic fatigue and feel suddenly conscious of your limitations – it can be very helpful to turn to nature for help. What never ceases to delight us both is how beautifully she responds to our demands.

We have always believed that health is fundamentally of our own making and that the responsibility for it lies in our own hands. When we find ourselves feeling under par, coming down with a cold for example, we know that somehow, whether knowingly or not, we have been living carelessly so that now our bodies are in need of clearing out. We believe, as the long tradition of natural medicine teaches, that a cold is a way of doing just that. So, instead of stuffing ourselves with antihistamines and aspirin, we try to go *with* the process, letting nature work through us. This means that everything we do – from fasting or eating only fruit to taking vitamin C (the master detoxifier) – is designed to encourage the rapid and efficient elimination of waste. The wonderful thing about it is that by going with nature, we avoid so much of the suffering we would have if we tried to block her. The colds that threaten to overcome us seldom take hold at all and a few days on all-raw foods plus vitamin C leaves us feeling far better than we did before the first sign of a sniffle.

In this section we explore some of the simple, natural helpers for maintaining high-level health – from nutritional supplements and life style changes for helping premenstrual syndrome to large doses of exercise as a way of bringing you in touch with reality in all its facets. You will find remedies which we use often and from which we and others have gained tremendous benefit. Included here is our Inner Sweep regime – a way of eating which we follow every few months for a week or ten days to clear away the mental and physical cobwebs and help the body regenerate itself. There may even be one or two things in this section which you have never heard of but which we believe are very important in keeping the body really well, such as how to maintain the balance and quality of micro-organisms in the colon.

And what about medical care? Of course, it is vital when you really need it. We would never suggest that anybody try to deal with serious illness on their own. But what is wonderful about the help that nature can give is that most often, when you listen to the messages she is sending you, you yourself can take action long before serious illness is allowed to develop.

WOMANWISE

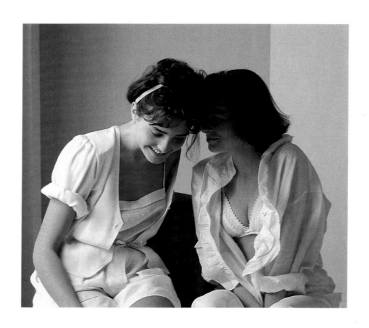

PRE-MENSTRUAL SYNDROME

Pre-menstrual syndrome, with its bloating, depression, irritability, fatigue and all the rest, is *not* something 'normal' with which you have to suffer, month in, month out. Some of the most resistant cases of PMS turn around when you change your diet, alter your living habits and use certain nutritional supplements. There is a great deal you can do yourself to make your periods less of a problem.

A way of eating in which 75 per cent of your foods are raw is the single most effective thing you can do to help period problems. Avoid too much salt – a prime troublemaker for PMS. Cook imaginatively, using herbs and spices, and steer clear of salty foods such as smoked fish, bacon, salted peanuts and processed foods. Regular vigorous aerobic exercise is another excellent antidote for PMS, because it both improves your mental and emotional state by altering brain chemistry and it encourages the body's metabolic processes to function smoothly. Don't drink tea or coffee. They can cause irritability, sleeplessness and stomach upsets, and make PMS worse. Opt instead for a grain beverage or herb teas. Stress tends to trigger PMS symptoms as well, so meditate regularly. This not only alters your biochemistry, it helps you manage the stressors in your life better.

● **Supplementary benefits** Women with PMS tend to have low magnesium levels in their blood. This is a mineral which is easily depleted by stress, a poor diet of processed foods, drinking too much tea, coffee or alcohol, smoking or eating too few fresh, raw leafy vegetables. This is one of the reasons why the high-raw way of eating is so effective in treating PMS. Supplements of vitamin B6 are often helpful against PMS, in part because B6 helps your body make use of magnesium in many of its vital processes and also because B6 helps correct hormone imbalances connected with menstrual difficulties. Zinc is another important nutrient which in supplemental form is useful for treating PMS. So is vitamin C and evening primrose oil. Here is what a typical anti-PMS nutritional formula looks like:

Magnesium aspartate	500 mg twice a day with meals
B6	10–30 mg three times a day with meals
Zinc citrate	15 mg twice a day with meals
Vitamin C	1–2 g three times a day
Evening primrose oil	1–2 500 mg capsules three times a day

This kind of formula is best taken for two or three months, after which many women find they only need take it for a 10–day period each month starting five days before a period. With improved nutrition, better stress management and the avoidance of coffee and tea, after a few months of this kind of nutritional support many women find their periods can remain trouble-free without taking any extra supplements whatever.

COUNTERING PILL PROBLEMS

Taking the contraceptive pill can also result in physical and emotional health problems because the hormones which it contains make high demands on many important nutrients. In fact, taking the Pill in many ways mimics the effect of pregnancy, which is why some women on it experience unpleasant symptoms such as water retention, queasy stomach and tender breasts. Even those who remain symptom-free still need extra nutritional support from nutrients such as zinc, folic acid, B6, vitamin C and B12 as well as some of the amino acids. Unfortunately, too few doctors as yet are

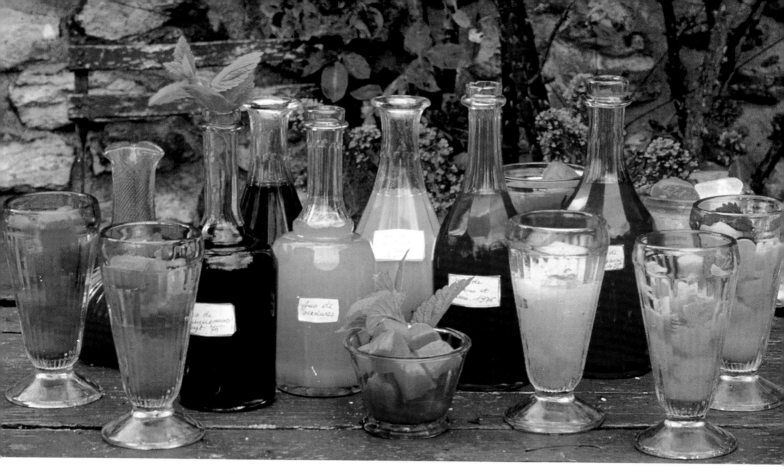

successfully as a part of treatment for manic depression and vascular diseases. There are now available some excellent formulas of phosphatidyl choline – the best come in the form of enriched lecithin granules which you can sprinkle onto cereals, soups or salads or mix in fruit juice. They provide as much choline as 12 high-potency lecithin capsules and are quite pleasant tasting.

RAW START
Although we eat a lot of raw foods, when we do eat a cooked meal we are always very careful to begin with something raw – usually a small salad. This is so we avoid a phenomenon called 'digestive leucocytosis'.

This rather grand phrase describes what happens in the gut when you eat cooked or processed food. For some reason, the cooked food in the mouth acts as a trigger to leucocytes (white blood cells) in the body, which rush to the intestines as if to defend the body from invasion. This means that there are fewer leucocytes in the rest of the body to protect it from disease. When you eat raw food, digestive leucocytosis does not occur. Similarly, if you eat raw food followed by cooked, you can also avoid the process.

If we are at a restaurant we will order a raw appetizer, such as melon, crudités or a mixed salad. If none of these are available, and we know ahead of time it will be difficult to start raw, then we will eat an apple on the way to the restaurant. By starting raw, you not only avoid digestive leucocytosis, you also stimulate enzymatic secretions and improve your digestion and assimilation of the meal to come.

BREATHE YOUR APPETIZER
Before you begin your meal – wherever you are – try taking 10 slow deep breaths. This is a wonderful trick to relax you and to prepare your body to enjoy its meal. You will also find that breathing seems quite literally to fill you up so you need to eat less. This is a godsend for anyone who wants to lose some weight, but seems ravenously hungry all the time. You can also use the magic 10 breaths between meals when you feel hunger pangs coming on. It is worth remembering that there are reports of people living entirely on air and water without food for months at a time. In general we eat far more than we need for optimum health, so breathe your appetizer and eat your entrée.

RELAX IN AN AIR BATH
Of all the nature cure treatments, the air bath is the simplest. It involves removing all your clothing and allowing fresh air to circulate around your body for a few minutes. It is believed that exposing the body in this way for only 10 minutes can increase metabolism temporarily by as much as 50 per cent. Certainly it makes sense to give our entire skin surface a chance to breathe unrestricted by clothing. The easiest way to incorporate an air bath into your daily routine is to strip down while you do your morning or evening toilet. Make sure you open a window in the bathroom so that there is fresh air. If you need to turn on a heater in the room do, although cool air on your body for a few minutes can have a positive, stimulating and strengthening effect.

Help Time

CRACKING COLDS & FLU

The common cold is one of the most frustrating and persistent illnesses there is. Most people just resign themselves to a yearly or twice yearly bout of sniffles, sore throats, coughs and aches. But we believe that no one need suffer a full-blown cold. As soon as you feel the slightest twinge of something coming on, go with the elimination process and be symptom-free within a day or two.

TO EAT OR NOT TO EAT?

We find it's best to starve a fever *and* a cold. When you're sick, your body is burning up wastes and fighting off an invasion, so it doesn't need to cope with digesting heavy meals too. At the first signs of a cold or flu, we stop eating and go onto a sustenance diet of apples and/or grapes. It's particularly important to avoid milk products, as they are highly mucus-forming and will only contribute to blocked sinuses. Eating fruit or drinking fluids is beneficial but it is essential that you choose the right ones.

The myth that you need glass after glass of orange juice to fight a cold is simply untrue. If you do drink fruit juice it should be freshly pressed (preferably not citrus), ideally combined with vegetable juice, which has a lower sugar content. If you only have packaged juice available, such as grape or apple, then dilute the fruit sugar by mixing it half-and-half with water.

A hot drink can be helpful in fighting a cold because it raises the temperature of the throat where viruses lurk. Viruses favour a cool climate, which is why going out in the cold when you have already caught a bug can make things worse. Choose a healing herb tea, such as camomile, lemon balm, peppermint or vervain, with a little honey. Our favourite 'hot toddy' is ginger tea. Grate 2 tablespoons (30 ml) of fresh ginger root and boil it in a small saucepan with 2–3 cups (16–24 fl oz/450–675 ml) of water for about 10 minutes. You can also add cloves and cinnamon to the boiling water. Remove the saucepan from the heat and strain the tea into a cup. Add a squeeze of lemon and a teaspoon of honey to sweeten, and sip slowly. If you can stand it, add $\frac{1}{8}$ teaspoon (0.5 ml) of cayenne pepper to the drink. This is one of the best spices for clearing sinuses and lungs.

As far as vitamins and mineral supplements go, we increase our intake of vitamin C as much as 10 or 20 g spread out through the day. We will also take about 100,000 IU of vitamin A for several days. Perhaps the most remarkable nutritional supplement for fighting a cold, however, is zinc lozenges. Zinc is needed in a diet for a strong immune system. Reseachers have found that the most effective way of taking zinc is in the form of a lozenge which is allowed to dissolve in the mouth. Scientists believe that the lozenges work so well because the zinc ions come into direct contact with the cold viruses in the respiratory tract and inhibit viral replication. We ourselves have found that sucking on zinc lozenges can instantaneously relieve a tickly throat.

Another helpful remedy for a tickly throat is to gargle with a strong solution of vitamin C (ascorbic acid) in water – 1 teaspoon (5 ml) to a glass. The herbal remedy is gargling with a strong cup of cooled red sage tea. Our friend Dr Gordon Latto swears by the garlic cure for a sore throat. Place a small clove of garlic (unpeeled) between your cheek and lower jaw and leave it there for half an hour or so. Garlic is nature's answer to antibiotics and this cure works a treat.

INDUCING FEVER

Fever is one of the greatest blessings in curing a bad cold or flu. It is the body's natural defence against viral or bacterial invasion. White blood cells respond to such an attack by producing a substance called pyrogen (meaning 'heat-producing') which signals the brain to raise the body's temperature to the point where the bacteria and viruses can no longer exist. As long as a fever doesn't go too high, it is a good thing.

Raising the body temperature in different places can be helpful in fighting off a viral infection. The archetypal image of a common cold victim is a person sitting in a chair with his feet in a basin of steaming water. The hot foot bath is actually one of the most useful techniques for treating colds or flu. It induces sweating, decreases internal congestion and relieves headache. It's important that you are well wrapped up. The feet should be immersed in the water up to the ankles for about 15 minutes. You should top up the bowl with hot water so that it remains as warm as you can stand it. After 15 minutes rinse your feet quickly with cold water, dry them well and wrap them in warm socks.

Applying heat directly to the nostrils and bronchial tubes can also be helpful for clearing sinuses and easing a cough. For nasal passages try inhaling a warm water and sea salt solution (1 teaspoon [5 ml] salt to a small bowl of water). Do one nostril at a time and spit the water out when it gets to the back of the throat. Again, the warmth of the water is helpful for combatting viruses in the nasal passages.

Another helpful hydrotherapy technique is inhaling steam. Pour boiling water into a large basin and cover your head with a towel. Breathe in the steam for several minutes. A peppermint tea sachet or some mint leaves added to the water are also beneficial. At the same time you will be giving yourself a facial. Cleanse your face well after steaming and put on your favourite moisturizer. Your open pores will drink it up!

MIND OVER VIRUS
Doctors and psychologists acknowledge a psychosomatic component to many illnesses, including colds.

Researchers experimenting with the psychological contribution to the development of colds have found that people who are withdrawn from friends, participate in few hobbies or who have recently experienced a drastic life change are more susceptible to colds and flu than their outgoing, friendly, happy counterparts. Your state of mind is important in resisting illness or recovering from it.

When you find yourself coming down with a cold it is worth asking, 'Why am I sick?' Usually it is a sign that your body is objecting to the way you are living, on a physical, emotional or even spiritual level. Get to the root of the problem and make changes for the better – put your health first and everything else will fall into place. Once you are happy and treating your body well, you will resist disease and, even if you are exposed to viruses, you will not be brought down by them.

EASING ACHES AND PAINS

● **General aching** is often the result of a build-up of toxic matter in the tissues. This can have many different causes. It can be something you've eaten (often the cause of migraine headache), the result of metabolic wastes from anaerobic exercise (muscle aches), headaches from environmental pollution or simply waste products from poor sleep and too much stress. Whatever the cause, it is important to stop and listen to your body whenever you feel pain. Taking pain-killers is not really helpful because they only relieve the surface symptoms. The amino acid DL-phenylalanine can be useful as a pain reliever.

● **Headaches** often arise from muscle tensions and poor posture, commonly as a result of leaning over a desk at work. If you have the opportunity, the best thing to do is to lie down on your back with your knees bent and a book such as a telephone directory under your head. Then practise deep breathing exercises. If you are out and about, try a quick head massage to

relieve tension. Begin at the base of the skull and apply pressure with your thumbs placed on either side of your spine in line with the bottom of your ears for about a minute. Then massage your scalp with your fingertips, beginning at the centre at your hairline and gradually working back. For sinus headache press your thumbs into the inner corners of the eyebrows, just beneath the brow bone, then massage down the sides of the nose and across the cheeks, draining away the congestion.

● **Allergy headaches** can be a symptom of food allergy or sensitivity. If you get a headache shortly after a meal, a food allergy is extremely likely. Remember what you have eaten and try to trace the 'suspect' food. The most common allergens are milk products, wheat and chocolate. One way to test for an allergen is to take your pulse, then eat a suspect food and then take your pulse again a few minutes later. If it has risen by 10 or more beats per minute it is likely you have a sensitivity to that food and should avoid

it to see if this makes you feel better.

● **Migraine headache** is a very intense head pain, usually located on one side of the head and often accompanied by nausea, mental aberration, blurred vision and even vomiting. The symptoms are caused by the expansion and contraction of blood vessels within the brain and skull. This contraction of blood vessels produces a squeezing effect on the brain. Migraine can develop from emotional, mental or physical stress or as a result of food allergy. The most common food troublemakers in descending order are: chocolate, dairy products, citrus fruits, alcohol, fatty fried foods, onions, pork, tea, coffee and seafood. Although conventional medicine does not recognize a cure for migraine, Dr Max Gerson and others have achieved tremendous success treating the illness with a high-raw diet.

● **Muscle aches** are often due to the build-up of lactic acid in the muscles as a result of anaerobic exercise.

One of the best treatments is to lie for 10 minutes in a warm bath to which a handful of Epsom salts, which help to draw out the wastes, has been added. If you can find someone to give you a good all-over body massage, it can be a great relief to aching muscles.

● **Backache** can be very debilitating. Whether it's caused by toxic wastes from eating the wrong foods, from poor posture, lifting heavy objects, sleeping awkwardly, etc., there are many things you can do to help. By focussing your attention on the painful area you can concentrate on relaxing the muscles out of spasm and breathing away the pain. If you regularly suffer from back pain, it may be because your back muscles are permanently tense and so tend to store toxins rather than eliminate them. As muscles work in opposite pairs, a permanently tight back will mean a slack stomach. Tone up your abdominal muscles, then your back muscles will be able both to relax and contract, and so release stored wastes.

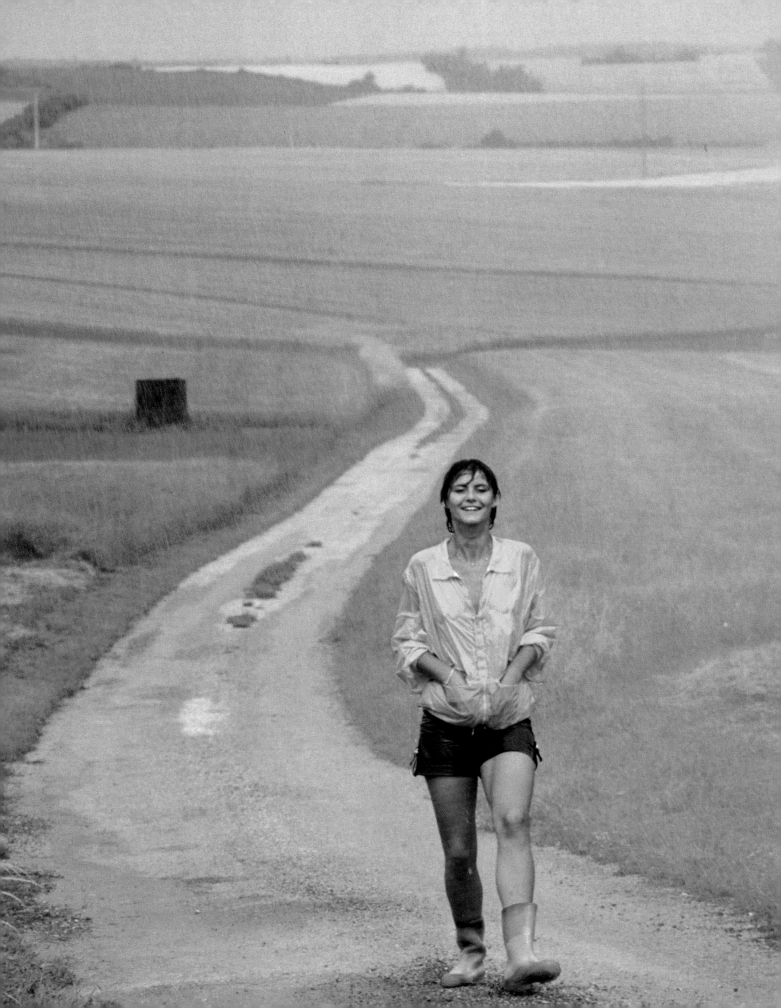

SELF TIME

Superlative health and lasting beauty need not be the province of a privileged few. They are within grasp of most of us. The only catch is you have to know where to look for them. For they are not to be found in books on exercise and diet, neither do they come in expensive jars of cosmetics – although all of these things can have a part to play in creating glowing skin and a high-energy life style for yourself. It is just that what you can get from these 'externals' really comes *second*. What comes *first* is something most of us tend badly to neglect, either because we are too busy or because it makes us uncomfortable: looking *inside*.

To be beautiful, to break the barriers for energy and good looks, you must be what you are. For what you are is far more interesting, vital and attractive than anything or anyone you might pretend to be. And what you need to be complete, beautiful, healthy, happy and fulfilled is not 'out there', 'one day', or 'if only I had . . .', it is already *here* – inside you. It does not need to be bought, seduced or copied. It simply needs to be discovered within you and then set free.

Every woman is in reality two women. The first, the *outer* woman, is a collection of physical characteristics, habits of speech and movement, and ways of thinking and of expressing herself. The outer part is the result of past experience, conditioning and values – either your own or, more often, those given you by your family, educational background and society, plus a great many preconceived ideas you have about who you are and what you can and can't do. This outer woman comes in many different forms. She may be conventionally attractive, plain, sexy, dynamic, withdrawn, aggressive, apparently assured or terribly uncertain about herself.

For each woman there is also an inner counterpart – an individual *self* which is utterly unique. A stable centre of strength and growth, this inner self sees the world in her own way, has her own needs, desires and her own brand of creativity, and is a law unto herself. It is this self which holds the power to create, change, build and transform your health and good looks for the better. The outer woman – how you look and dress and how rich in energy and wellness your life is – fundamentally depends upon what the self creates. And it is here that the make-up and the clothes and the jewellery have a real part to play as delightful and amusing tools with which to play the creative game of self-decoration – not as heavy uniforms of other people's expectations or status symbols.

This section of *Time Alive* is all about exploring the inner you. It deals with the many things which can be helpful in coming to know the power of the self and then finding authentic expression for it in your life. Doing this involves transformation. It can get you involved in a process of development which can not only be tremendously exciting, but can release enormous energy and joy and quite literally rejuvenate and regenerate your whole body. Sometimes this process can also be quite hard, but it is enormously rewarding. And this transformative process lies at the very core of the *Time Alive* journey towards energy and lasting good looks.

RUN TO REALITY

We run. Not that there is anything special about running. But in the modern world, in which life tends to be physically unchallenging and it is all too easy for us to sit back like indolent toads and watch television, we *need* the power of discipline which it brings. Of course, discipline is not popular in twentieth-century Western life. It is one of those 'no-no' words. For most of us prefer some kind of passive pleasure.

Many a joke has been made about the man or woman who, every time he or she feels an urge to exercise, lies down until it passes. After all, who would want to sweat and smell and be seen to be puffing away at something when you can remain cool and unfettered, and let the rest make fools of themselves?

We would. We would because we have learned the hard way that only through a certain amount of self-discipline (and neither of us has much naturally) can one find freedom. Only if you take an active part in your life can you reap the rewards of being fully alive.

We don't run because it is good for us. And neither of us is a good runner. We are never going to win a marathon and we are never going to move with that wonderful sense of grace you occasionally see in someone who is. Yet we continue to sweat. We continue to get up every morning – even if we feel exhausted, it's raining and we would rather turn over and spend another hour in bed – put on our dirty running shoes and head for the road. Why? Because the alternative – that of being simply the passive observer of life, someone who doesn't give of himself – would be all too easy for us both. Because both of us by nature are quite passive and lazy and we know ourselves well. And, most important of all, because, having done it over and over again throughout the months and years, we know that running, like any form of aerobic exercise which you do day after day, releases energy which we can use in other areas of our lives.

It also teaches us a lot about ourselves and about living. Hours on the road have shown us both that we are capable of achieving things we never thought we could accomplish. Through the sweat and the resistance, the successes and the failures, we have learned a lot about our strengths and our limitations. And we have rediscovered that sense of play, of doing something for its own sake, which children have, but adults too often lose completely. There is something quite

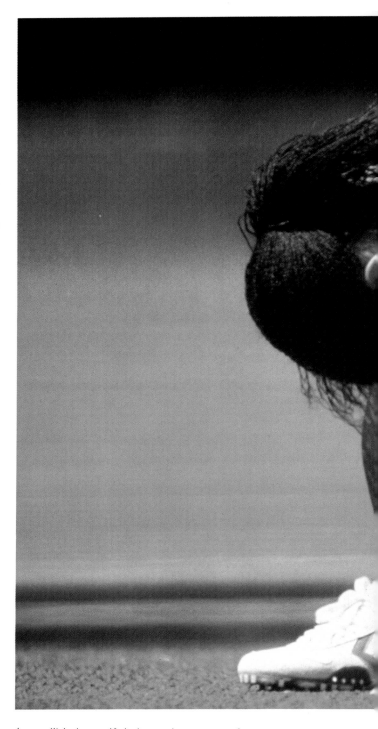

incredibly beautiful about the sense of oneness you can feel with every living thing as your body moves steadily over the earth. Sometimes, suddenly, there isn't any you – there is only life and you are part of it.

Both of us have strong tendencies to quit, to walk away from something when the going gets rough. Running has also taught us that we don't *have* to – that we can instead choose to stick it out and persevere even when things get difficult. And it has brought us face to face with our own limitations. We hope it has

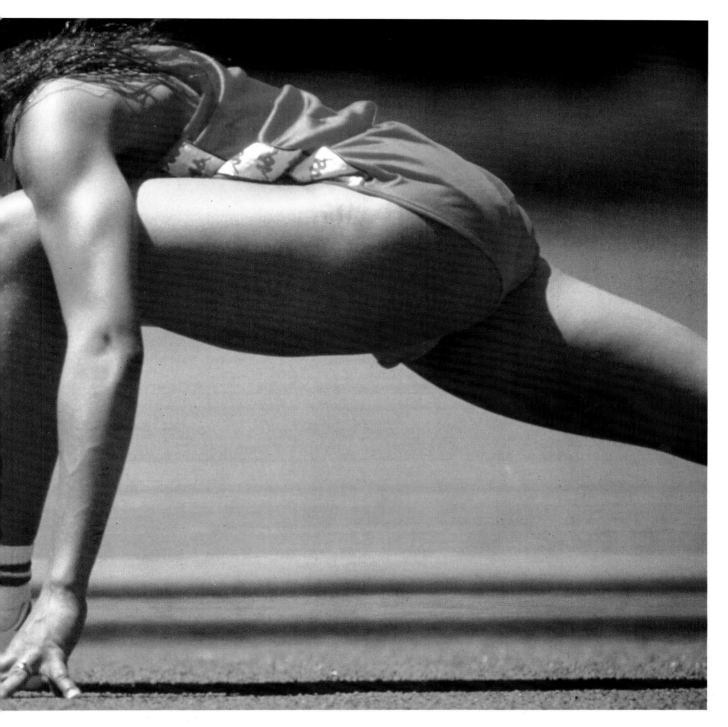

also taught us to be a little more tolerant of the limitations of others. In short, each morning as we head out to run our miles we come face to face with reality. Sometimes that reality is hard and ugly. Sometimes it is wonderful beyond description. But it is *our* reality and it has to be lived not only now, but all through every changing day of our lives. In a very simple, practical way, running helps us do that.

These are some of the reasons, quite apart from all the physical benefits you can get from exercise, that we urge *you* to take up your own form of exercise, whatever it may be – from walking to rowing or cycling or dancing. Always check your heart rate to make sure you are exercising at a safe level for your current level of fitness (see p. 20). (You will be amazed to find how quickly you become more fit.) Whatever activity you choose, and whatever your present state of fitness, do it, make it *yours* and follow it regularly. It will transform your energy levels and expand your consciousness. It is the best road to freedom we have ever found.

CURE YOURSELF LAUGHING

Laughter and humour are much needed in the over-serious world of health and beauty which can make you neurotic about what to eat and not to eat. It is a world which tends to measure health not as joyous energy and creativity, but in terms of cholesterol levels, blood pressure and sedimentation rates.

The irony of it all is that, according to the latest research into the mind–body relationship, a life which sparkles with laughter is not only good for you because it *feels* good. It can also help look after the state of your blood pressure, immune system and cholesterol levels – some researchers believe far better than high-powered medical care drugs. Drugs, after all, can have deeply worrying side-effects. The worst of laughter's side-effects is joy.

When we laugh we shed feelings of judgement, self-pity and blame. Our perception shifts and we come to know another level of consciousness. Laughter deepens your breathing, expands blood vessels, heightens circulation (bringing more oxygen to your cells), increases the secretion of hormones beneficial to your body, speeds tissue-healing and helps stabilize bodily functions. A new philosophy is emerging from studies carried out in France and Canada by philosopher André Moreau on the notion that we should seek in all philosophical teachings the keys for releasing innate human tendencies towards humour, laughter and positive energies. Known as 'jovialisme', it advocates the practice of smiling as a free expression of human vitality and creativity. We are much in favour of it. We spend a good quarter of the time we're together laughing.

Meanwhile hospitals both in the United States and Europe are even prescribing laughter in the form of Jerry Lewis' and the Marx Brothers' films, humorous books and any other simple triggers to put patients into a blissful state of spontaneous giggles.

LIFE ON THE FLIP SIDE
The way that emotions and health are closely related has been investigated for many years. The scientific press is full of papers which show the way that negative emotions, such as anger, resentment, fear and despair, are major factors in the development of serious illness, from cancer to coronary heart disease. Scientists have charted direct pathways between mind and immunity via anatomical connections that link the brain directly to organs such as the spleen and the thymus gland. They have also shown that hormonal secretions induced by emotions and thought patterns create a second pathway between mind and body which is carried in the blood, and there is strong evidence that excess adrenalin from high levels of stress can significantly depress your body's immune system. But until recently most of the focus of mind–body research has been on the *negative*.

Now, thanks to the new fascination with laughter, many scientists are beginning to investigate the biochemical changes brought about by *positive* emotions and to encourage their use as tools for health and healing. Researchers now find that laughter, relaxation, meditation and hope not only produce beneficial changes such as lowered heart rate and breathing, they can even improve the way your body responds to stress hormones and bring about a shift in your perception of potentially stressful situations so you can look on them as challenges rather than as insurmountable problems – a vital attitude in preserving and enhancing the health of your mind and body.

HUMOUR MELTS THE EGO
One of the very best things of all about laughter is that it breaks through the tendency each of us has to take ourself and our values too seriously. It breaks down the roles we play and liberates the self locked within. It is our tendency to identify with our own self-created image, fears, beliefs and assumptions that takes us away from the joy which we believe is *normal* for each of us to feel. Give yourself a chance to laugh even if it means watching an old Marx Brothers' film on TV or having a silly evening with friends. It will make you more alive, healthier and more beautiful.

LEARN TO LAUGH
● Seek out and spend time with people who make you laugh – often.

● Look for books which make you laugh and keep a file of cartoons and magazine articles which you can share with your friends.

● Rediscover the art of being silly – like a child. Maybe join a drama class where they do improvisation, or make friends with children who still remember how to laugh and play, and let them be your teachers.

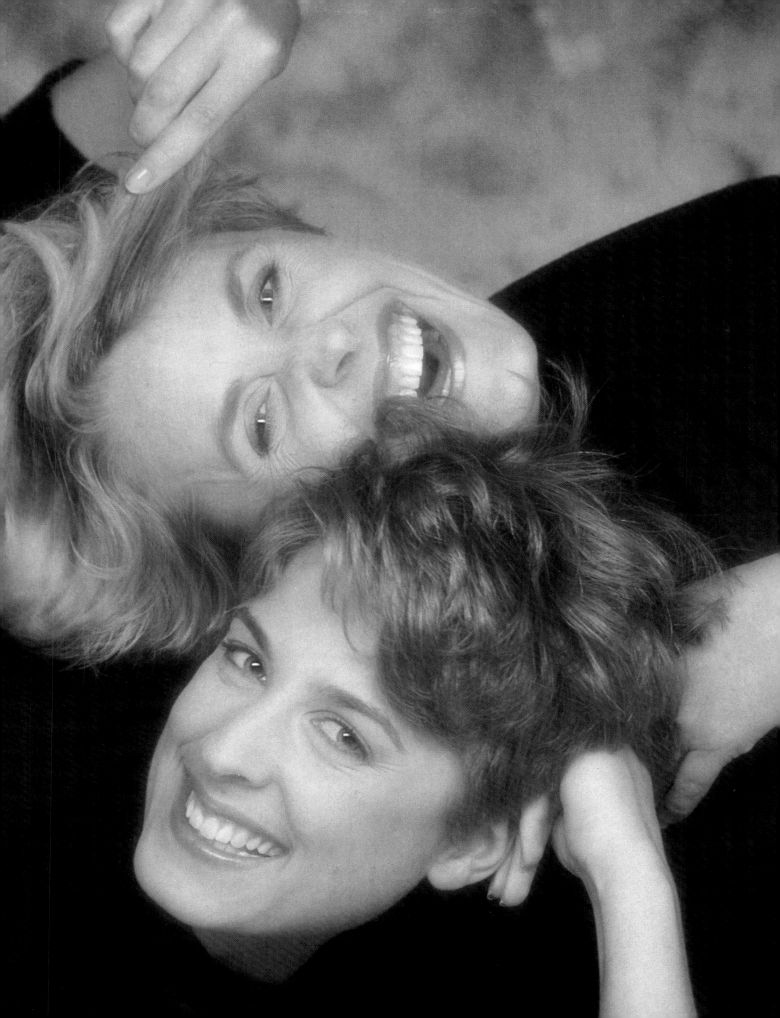

EMOTIONAL ECOLOGY

What is your emotional life like? A dazzling technicolour circus in which you, the trapeze artist, find yourself frequently in the net? A bleak desert where everything exciting goes on not *here*, where you are, but somewhere else? A roller coaster you're on and can't get off as it takes you relentlessly to the heights and depths along the track while you hold on helpless? Or are you one of the lucky few? Is your emotional expression like a finely woven tapestry of lights and darks which intermingle and complement each other in perfect harmony?

Everybody's way of expending emotional energy is different – as different as the amount of energy we have to expend. And despite the 'happily ever after' myths propagated by romantic novels, life is a series of emotional ups and downs, not a continuous blissful turn-on. When you feel yourself well stocked with emotional energy, say on holiday or when you've just started a new romance, there is no end to the excitement and expansiveness you can feel. But when your emotional reserves are ebbing, almost anything can seem irritating, boring, purposeless and dull.

How well you cope with the natural emotional ups and downs we all experience depends a lot on how able you are, through a little simple introspection, to modulate the dramatic ebb and flow of your emotional energy and to learn the art of fine-tuning your own responses to things. For emotional energy is part of your energy as a whole. Its regeneration is governed by the same rules of balance and it responds to the same gentle persuasion. Hoard your emotions in order to protect yourself and you'll end up feeling bleak and lifeless – feeling your energy unable to flow freely. Expend them unwisely and you'll be left flat, with that awful sense of having burned yourself out and feeling nothing at all any more. Balance is the real key.

ARE YOU A GIVER OR A TAKER?
These are two fundamental emotional styles. Both have their pitfalls. This may surprise you since everybody tends to praise the 'givers'. They are the ones who are always there offering help, who jump when anything needs to be done, who have a great deal of sympathy for others and who seem sometimes to draw on endless emotional reserves to keep going after the rest of us are worn out. You can recognize a giver behind many different masks. He or she is the life of the party, the loving mother or the considerate friend who is for ever providing a sympathetic ear, a bed for the night, a meal. The giver can be a tower of strength on whom everybody seems to rely.

And giving is good. There is a kind of natural law – the more you give, the more you receive. It's a law every giver instinctively knows, and it would seem at first glance that givers have all the luck. But look again. Behind that cheerful mask of generosity you will often find a deep need to be liked – a person who is not very sure of himself and who gains his sense of worth not from what he *is* but from what he *does* for people or from the way in which they respond to him. In fact, the givers are a complex lot. For mixed in with that wonderful and quite genuine generosity you may also find a great deal of subtle manipulation and several implicit 'bargains': 'I will do for you if you will only . . .'. These are, alas, bargains which are all too seldom fulfilled. They lead many givers to experience debilitating feelings of resentment – the sense that they have squandered too much of their emotional strength. They have given their all, but nobody seems to appreciate them.

PROS AND CONS FOR THE TAKING
Like the archetypal dragon who glowers in its cave protecting its precious treasure, despite their attempts to amass even more emotional wealth for themselves, the counterparts of these givers – the 'takers' – never allow their emotional jewels to sparkle in the sunlight. They have trouble sharing. Their emotional life tends to be limited, bleak, rather empty. They, more than anybody, tend to be plagued by the sense that everything exciting is happening somewhere else. Because, well, everybody knows that being a taker is not nearly as good as being a giver. But isn't it? In fact, there can be some pretty positive things about the kind of emotional restraint and self-centredness which is second nature to a taker. For one thing, takers seldom waste themselves in emotional bargaining. They are often more honest than their emotionally effusive relatives and – best of all – it is often the takers who are able to get things done, to accomplish the goals they set for themselves. For they may seem stingy and not so much fun to be around, but they never squander emotional energy like the givers do. Many of the greatest writers, artists and

composers have been emotionally stingy people. It is as if they were able to save up this energy and turn it into something beautiful.

BALANCE IS THE KEY
In fact, there is no such thing as a pure giver or taker. They are only emotional styles. And far from being mutually exclusive, they beautifully complement each other. To make the best use of our emotional energy each of us needs some of the characteristics of both. We need to know when to let go and to allow the feeling to flow – when to give without expectation. But we must also never allow giving to become a compulsion so that we can reserve the kind of creative energy that is central to fulfilling our own goals.

MEET THE POSITIVES AND THE NEGATIVES
One of the best ways to begin taking stock of how effectively you use your emotional reserves is to take a look at the company you keep. Are well over half of your friends chosen from active, energetic, cheerful people who keep you thinking about new ideas and have you trying new things? If so, you probably have few problems with emotional depletion. These people are the 'positives' of emotional energy. Because they tend to be self-sufficient and are not wrapped up in themselves, they seldom deplete your own energy reserves.

Spending too much time in the company of the 'negatives', however, can quite literally drain you of emotional strength. Most of us know the negatives only too well. They are constantly complaining or feeling hopeless about something. They delight in telling you all about their latest illness or heartbreak and they seem to derive a certain masochistic pleasure in their romantic hopes and dreams being shattered. Some of these negatives can be quite charming and intelligent people, and if you are a real giver yourself, with a lot of emotional energy to spare, then having a close relationship with one or two can do you both good. Indeed, the negatives bring a lot of interesting shadows into a world which may be too dynamic and high-key. But they are also basically 'downers'. They don't stimulate, uplift and energize as positives do, despite whatever dark fascination they can sometimes elicit from those around them.

Unless you yourself are a *superpositive*, with lots of emotional energy to spare, leave these fascinating

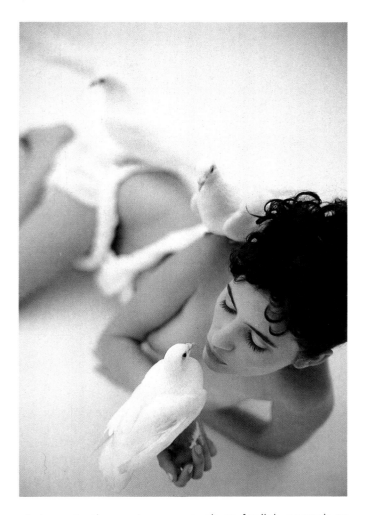

drainers to those strong enough or foolish enough to deal with them. Learn to say to the complaining person as he is just about to tell you how bad things are, 'Look, friend, I'm just a little wiped out myself right now – let's talk about it later.' You may think you are being unsympathetic or unkind, but in reality you can be doing something good for him as well as yourself.

PAUSE BEFORE YOU PROMISE
Another helpful trick for energy conservation is to think ahead before you make promises. A lot of natural givers are for ever saying things like, 'Do come and stay for a few days whenever you like' or 'I'd be happy to help out with the party, what can I do?' before they stop to think just what kind of commitment in time and energy such promises imply. You can find yourself with some work to finish, people dropping in and expecting a bed and a sick friend in need of tending, all at once at the end of a long week when you need a few days to yourself. This is where you can learn something from the takers. They never make off-hand offers, no matter how generous and spontaneous they're feeling. They also don't suffer the feelings of fatigue, inadequacy and resentment when too many of these promises are called up all at once.

MIND POWER

Every one of us has more potential for health, happiness, self-expression, energy and good looks than we ever make use of. *Time Alive* is about becoming aware of that potential and discovering techniques to help tap it. Although there are many tools to help you towards self-fulfilment – good food, exercise, stress control, beauty techniques, etc. – we believe that by far the most important of all is learning to use the full power of your own mind.

GET THINGS IN PERSPECTIVE

What do you do when trouble strikes? Everybody has those days when everything seems to go wrong all at once – you burn the toast, stain your blouse, pick up the telephone to hear some very rude neighbour complaining about last night's party, go to work and find a pile of tedious things to do sitting on your desk and by five o'clock find yourself feeling depleted, angry and miserable. It's time to gain some perspective on your predicament, separate the really important things from those that are nothing but little niggling problems, and deal with one thing at a time. Never let that awful old saying 'Why me?' gain ground in your consciousness. Do the best you can, bit by bit, and don't allow yourself to worry fruitlessly about things over which you have little control. In fact, one of the most depleting of all influences on our emotional reserves is just such worry. It saps strength and gets you into a kind of vicious circle of misery which only further depletes your energy.

At the end of the day, take time to relax, retreat and retire. Forgive yourself for not being perfect and treat yourself kindly so you can recuperate. If you find you are anxious still, try tidying a drawer of your desk – gently and just for fun. Straightening out the arrangement of physical things in your external world can have the most amazing effect on ordering your inner feelings and restoring energy levels and emotional balance. It's a trick many busy people under stress use often.

Of course, one of the best ways of all to make sure you never run out of emotional strength is to have such an abundance that little short of total disaster can possibly deplete it.

YOU ARE WHAT YOU THINK

Because we create our lives from thoughts, it is important that we think constructively. Unfortunately, most of us, without being aware of it, limit our possibilities for fulfilment by continually bombarding ourselves with negative thoughts. We all carry on some sort of internal conversation throughout the day. Usually, if we tune in and listen, we find that it is full of negative thoughts and self-doubts. Out of these negative thoughts arise our self-image and our sense of purpose and direction.

LOVE THYSELF

Whether you feel you are too fat, too thin, too short, too tall, too selfish, too sensitive, etc., in order to change you must begin by accepting yourself right now for what you are. Try this exercise: look at yourself in a mirror and repeat the words, 'I love and accept myself completely as I am', over and over in your head. And as you do, write down any blocks that seem to keep you from accepting yourself. You may feel stupid or ridiculous or embarrassed, but stick with the exercise and you will find that it begins to ring true.

POSITIVE AFFIRMATIONS

You can learn to programme your mind to bring about success and fulfilment in all areas of your life through positive affirmations. An affirmation is a phrase which can be silently thought, spoken aloud, written down, or all three. The great thing is that affirmations can be done any time and anywhere in one form or another. There are a few basic guidelines for contacting the appropriate part of your brain and evoking results. Once you understand them you can create your own affirmations to help you become all that you can be.

● **Present tense** The subconscious part of the brain only understands now – the present tense – so it is important to phrase your affirmation in the present tense. If you try the future tense ('I will be happy'), your goal will remain constantly out of your reach.

● **First person** The most powerful suggestions are those made in the first person. Remember, when you say 'I', you are including all of you and so helping to integrate and employ your entire being in your goals.

● **Positive** It is always better to make affirmations positive rather than negative. In other words, instead of saying 'I no longer overeat', say 'Everything I eat returns me to my ideal weight of . . .'.

● **Specific and realistic** Set yourself specific goals at first which are within your capabilities to achieve. Once

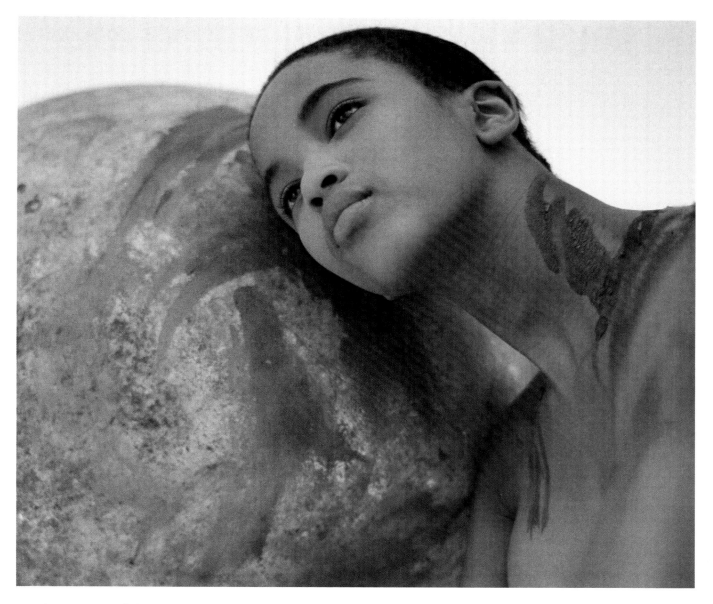

you have accomplished them you will be encouraged and can set more challenging goals. If you are trying to give up smoking, for instance, begin with the affirmation that you are cutting down the amount you smoke by half.

● **Short and simple** Keep affirmations as short and direct as possible. A concise, brief affirmation will have more impact than a long, wordy one.

● **Suspend disbelief** Try, while doing affirmations, to cast aside doubts and believe in the possibility of what you are saying.

● **Personally phrased** Make sure that you are happy with the wording of your affirmation. For each person the word choice may need to be slightly different. Feel free to change any of the affirmations we suggest to suit your own requirements.

● **All-encompassing** Remember that the affirmation can be used to transform any area of your life, from career and self-image to your relationships with others. Know that you have every right to be successful and happy and that your life is yours to create.

● **Some affirmations** Here are some of our favourite affirmations. We both like the written affirmations because for us they seem to solidify things. Other people prefer to repeat them silently in meditation, or even sing them. We find seven a useful number to work with. Repeat the affirmations in multiples of seven at a time.

Every day in every way I'm getting better and better.
I create my life and it is good.
I love and appreciate myself just as I am.
The more I give to others the more I have to give.
I have plenty of energy and I enjoy my work.
I have all the time I need to accomplish all I want.
It's okay for me to enjoy myself and have fun.

Self Time

JOURNEY TO THE CENTRE

The mind's depths are rarely plumbed in everyday life. In fact, scientists estimate that we usually use only a mere 10 per cent of our mental capacity – an unfortunate loss of potential. By expanding our consciousness and awareness and setting the power of imagination in motion, we can learn to draw upon the remaining reserves and use them to create and actualize our goals and dreams.

CREATIVE VISUALIZATION

The process is known as creative visualization or conscious dreaming. It is based on the principle that, in everything we do, a thought or an image always precedes an action. For example, the thought 'I will go and make dinner' or 'I am hungry' results in the meal. By using this principle we can programme our minds with positive and creative thoughts and images to bring about rewarding results. This is something which we have both worked with for a very long time.

That the mind is capable of influencing our lives and the world in which we live is only beginning to be appreciated. At cancer clinics throughout the world, doctors are starting to acknowledge the role of creative visualization in the seemingly miraculous 'spontaneous remission' of terminal patients. Patients are being taught to visualize their immune systems sending out white blood cells in armies to destroy malignant cells. The medical profession also acknowledges the power of the mind in its use of placebos. A placebo is an inert substance or procedure which a patient believes is a powerful therapeutic drug or technique and which often leads to a dramatic recovery from a serious physical illness. Such are the powers of the mind.

Conscious dreaming is a way of beginning to tap the powers of your mind in order to take control of your life and accept responsibility for what comes to you. It is done in a state of deep relaxation in which we are able to let go of the tensions, worries and doubts that normally plague us, and contact our deeper self. You can use conscious dreaming to improve all areas of your life, for instance, to give you more confidence and a better self-image, to improve your performance at work or in athletics, to intensify your healing abilities, to increase your creativity so that you express your talents with greater ease and even to gain insights into problems that vex you. It works on the principle that your

subconscious does not draw a distinction between an actual experience and a vivid mental image, so that your dreams can take on the weight of reality and eventually become part of and improve your conscious life.

DEEP RELAXATION

To begin the journey of self-discovery and transformation you need to relax deeply. Our favourite relaxation exercise was taught to us by a friend, Angela Farmer, a talented and dedicated teacher of yoga. It focusses on the breath to still the mind and body and is called the Total Breath. This complete exercise can be difficult to learn at first. Make yourself a tape of the instructions to use until they become second nature.

● **Making a relaxation tape** Record the following text for your relaxation exercise on tape, reading the instructions slowly, or have a friend with a soothing voice read them if you don't like the sound of your own voice. Ellipses (...) indicate that you should pause for several seconds to allow you to repeat an instruction in your mind or to visualize an image.

● **The Total Breath technique**

1 Begin by lying down on a carpet or blanket on the floor. (The firm surface of the floor is better than a bed because it allows your muscles to relax more deeply against it.) Make sure you are warm enough – cover yourself with a blanket if necessary. Place a rolled-up towel or blanket or book under your neck and head. (The size will depend upon the curvature of your neck.) Your head should be supported and your chin parallel to the floor. Make sure the phone is off the hook and that no one disturbs you. Lying on your back, bend your knees up and place your feet hip-width apart, comfortably near your buttocks. Bend your elbows and rest your palms on your abdomen.

2 Bring your awareness to the contact of your body with the ground. Notice where you touch the floor. Let yourself give up your entire weight to the floor so that you sink into it ... Imagine the earth embracing you from behind ... Let the breath flow through your body like water, gently easing away any tension ...

3 Once you have eased your back muscles on the floor, your spine will naturally lengthen out. Help this lengthening by putting your hands gently behind your head and easing your head and neck out. (You may have to readjust your head-rest.) ...

4 Instead of breathing, release your back to create a space and then wait for the breath to enter. This waiting is very important. It eliminates the sense of trying and doing which fills our everyday life. Trust that your breath will enter automatically. You need make no effort to breathe... As the breath enters, feel it rippling through the layers of muscle in your back and have the sense of 'it breathes me'...

5 Bring your awareness to the area where your legs attach to your pelvis and try to let go of any holding in your hips and pelvis. Don't try to move your legs, but imagine your knees being pulled gently up and away on a diagonal ... Consider the possibility of your legs floating away from your pelvis...

6 Now feel the weight of your pelvis against the floor. Imagine it as a hollow basin and let your belly and inner organs melt back into it ... Feel the bony part of the pelvis (the sacrum) spreading out on the floor as the breath comes in ... As the breath leaves, the spine lengthens out and the back relaxes back into the floor ...

7 Work slowly up the spine in this way. Take your awareness first to the lumbar area ... Check that it is not you *breathing*, but you *waiting*, *releasing*, *watching*, as the breath enters and leaves your body ... Observe as more and more layers of muscle give up their tensions ... Focus on the lower and middle back. When the breath enters the back of your rib-cage, remember that your ribs are only connected to the spine by cartilage and can expand to the sides to create more space for the breath ... Now take your awareness to your upper back. Allow the upper back to widen with the in-breath and lengthen with the out-breath ...

8 Notice any hardness and holding in the front ribs and chest, and allow them to soften ... The front of the body can sink back and be received by the back of the body ... Bring your attention to the shoulders and top of the chest. For most of us, a lot of worry, stress and fear are held here. See if you can gently soften in these areas, allowing the sternum (breastbone) to drop down and melt ... Let your shoulders gradually sink down towards the floor ... Imagine a point in the centre of your chest going through to the back between your shoulder-blades, and from this point see if you can allow the shoulders to drift apart ... The shoulder-blades can slide away from each other on the floor with the inhalation and rest separated on the out-breath ...

9 Let go of any tension in your throat and neck, and allow your head to float away from the rest of your body ... Let your hair flow away from your head ... Imagine your eyes as two pebbles dropping backwards into a pool of water ... Let the skin on your face become heavy and flow sideways and down towards your ears ...

10 Become aware of yourself as a whole ... Feel the gentle ebbing and flowing of the breath throughout your entire body ...

11 Allow yourself to enter the tranquil harbour of your mind and begin conscious dreaming ...

CONSCIOUS DREAMING

Explore a sanctuary within your mind to which you can return each time you do the conscious dreaming. Imagine yourself in a beautiful place. It may be a place from your past or entirely imaginary. Let yourself feel safe and at peace. Now evoke your dream. Picture your ideal self. If you want to lose weight, for instance, see yourself slim and happy, going about your everyday affairs. Try to see yourself as vividly as possible. Imagine other people you know responding positively to the ideal you. If you are sick, imagine yourself well again and doing your favourite things. If you have a problem, for example with a relationship that is not going well, or you need to make an important decision, quietly ask your inner self for advice. By taking the time to listen to your higher wisdom, you'll be surprised at how easily problems are resolved.

Successful conscious dreaming comes in both an active and a passive mode. You can create images and ideals for yourself actively, or you can take a receptive stance and allow images and thoughts to arise of their own accord. Both are important and can lead to valuable insights. At the end of each conscious dreaming session, conclude by saying to yourself, 'This or something better now happens to me for the total good of all concerned.' This phrase allows the possibility of the higher wisdom to work through your dreams.

Finally, open your eyes gradually and look around you for a few seconds. Slowly roll over onto one side and gently stand up. You can return to the conscious dream images throughout the day. By beginning to contact your inner self in this way, you will find that it becomes usefully integrated into your everyday life.

MIND-BENDING FRAGRANCES

Like music and meditation, aromatics can be used to alter your consciousness and deepen your awareness. Using environmental fragrances is also a delightful way to lift your mood and sharpen your mind. A cool whiff of neroli sets your brain racing. Sniffing white rose can nestle you down into the most enjoyable indolence. Immerse yourself in the rich warmth of the ambergris and, even if you are the most timid of creatures, you can begin to feel bold and daring.

The special substances that make all this possible are plant essences – the light, fine, almost ethereal essential oils taken from the roots, leaves, barks and flowers of plants in their prime of life. A plant essence plays an important role in the plant's growth to maturity, is for ever changing its chemical composition in the plant and is present in greatest quantities in young plants. Many experts in the use of plant essences believe that, in some way that no one has been able to identify, these substances contain much of the life force of the plant, including the basic characteristics of its leaves and flowers which give it a unique character, smell and ability to affect humans in specific ways.

Some plants, such as jasmine and rose, require hundreds of pounds of live flowers to produce even a tiny bottle of the essence. They are very expensive. Other oils, such as cinnamon and basil, are easily extracted and inexpensive. But you should know that the 'synthetic' version of a plant essence (in spite of the fact that its main constituents have been chemically reproduced) does not have the same effect on a person as the real thing. This is probably because the terpene alcohols, phenols and esters that make up these natural substances have a synergistic quality, that is, they work together to produce an effect greater than the sum of each working on its own.

MIND-BENDING MAGIC

Some natural therapists rely on many plant essences for their restorative and stimulating actions in treatments for skin and hair, as well as for combatting cellulite. They are also important constituents in many expensive face creams and lotions. But the way in which aromatic vibrations from essential oils can be used in your environment to alter mood and mind is something quite different from their therapeutic uses when mixed with carrier oils and spread on the skin in aromatherapy treatments. Oil of geranium, for instance, is a mild diuretic useful in aromatherapy for treating fluid retention, eczema and anxiety. But burn it as incense or let it diffuse into your environment as a fragrance, and it can make you act with uncharacteristic rashness – an effect quite separate from its therapeutic properties. Aromatherapy is a tool for healing. Aromatics belong to the realm of magic.

The best way to discover what its magic can do for you is to experiment with a few of the real essences. Start with six and then enlarge your repertoire as you get to know the quality and characteristics of each and as you discover those you particularly like. Because they are natural substances and highly volatile, they rapidly diffuse into the environment. They just as rapidly disappear or can be replaced by other fragrances.

When you choose essences and oils for burning, make absolutely sure that those you buy are natural. The current fascination with aromatherapy has led to the appearance of myriad poor-quality, so-called essential oils which are nothing of the kind. They are cheap chemical analogues and are currently being sold in chemists, department stores and speciality shops all over. Trying to use them for mind-bending is a grave mistake. They can actually make you feel quite sick, not to mention the unpleasant fact that they tend to infuse into a room and then imbed themselves in the carpets, curtains and furniture with the tenacity of a cheap perfume. Only real essential oils have mind-bending magic. But what a wonderful magic that can be!

USING AROMATICS FOR MIND-BENDING

● Put 30–50 drops of essential oil or oils into a 10 fl oz (2½ cup/112 ml)-size spray bottle filled with water. (The kind you use to spray plants is ideal.) Use this mixture as a room spray.
● Put 8–10 drops of essential oils on a small piece of cardboard and place it on a warm radiator.
● Put 5–10 drops of an essence on a small plate and put it on top of an Aga or wood-burning stove.
● Place a few drops of essential oils on a cotton or linen handkerchief and sniff it periodically. (This is particularly good if you are in a public place where the air is full of cigarette smoke or the room is stuffy.)
● Place 10–15 drops in a pan of simmering water. This will humidify the environment as well as scent it.

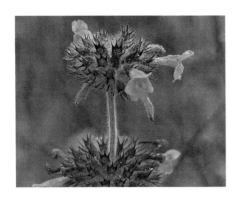

Basil Banishes fear and indecision

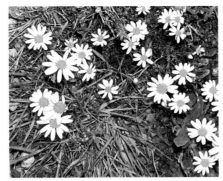

Camomile Against panic and hysteria

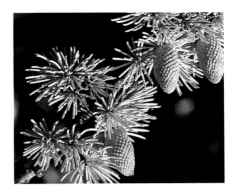

Cedar Heightens creativity

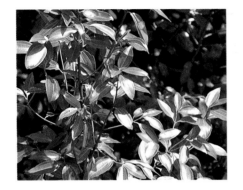

Cinnamon Natural stimulant

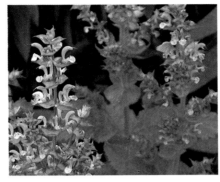

Clary sage Clears head after mental activity

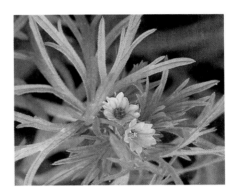

Geranium Anti-anxiety

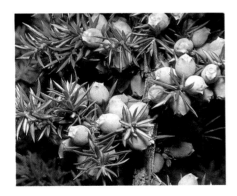

Juniper Improves concentration

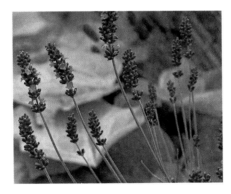

Lavender Calms irritability

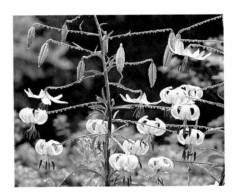

Lily Restores energy

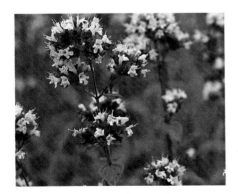

Marjoram Calms irritability, soothes panic

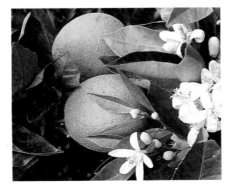

Neroli Anti-shock aid, heightens mental functions

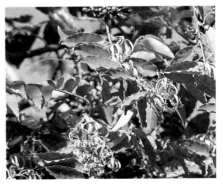

Ylang ylang Aphrodisiac, anti-depressant

Self Time

TIME OFF

Time off can mean a long weekend walking in the country or a month searching out the visual delights of Italy. It can even mean time away from home, working. Often these days any holiday you take can entail a long (sometimes) and uncomfortable (almost always) journey by plane. If you are going to get the most from travel, whether for work or pleasure, you will want to make it as easy as possible – particularly travel by plane. This means you need to think ahead.

PACK LIKE A PAUPER

Take little – about half of what you first lay out is usually just about right. Even experienced travellers tend to pack far too much and then end up slaves to their baggage. You need only the minimum quantities of underwear and socks, a night-dress, night-shirt or pyjamas, and two or three changes of clothes and your exercise kit to last you a fortnight in most places. And then, of course, if you are a runner, the inevitable muddy running shoes in their own plastic bag. Cosmetics? Great. But only small quantities. Make sure you can fit them into a little zip bag. You don't *need* that wonderful fuchsia eye-shadow 'just in case'. The colours you wear most of the time will do very well for both day and evening. And the clothes you choose, if possible, should be knits which don't crush or natural fabrics which do crush but look great that way. Put it all into a medium-size suitcase or sausage bag and leave room in the bag for expansion. What we often do on a trip is to slip another soft collapsible bag into the bottom of the one we are carrying. This means we can pull it out and fill it up with presents or things we see abroad which we can't resist buying. We invariably leave with one bag and return home with two.

JET-SETTING WITHOUT JET-LAG

For both of us, airplanes represent the absolute pits of misery. The air is foul, so are the smells, your skin gets dried out and your temper rises. And, if you are crossing more than a couple of time zones, you are probably going to have to wrestle with jet-lag, which befuddles the mind, depresses the spirit and exhausts the body.

The day before a long flight, eat only raw food – fruits and vegetables, sprouted seeds and grains. Do the same the day after. When you book your flight, or a few days before leaving, request a special meal of salad or fruit, or simply carry with you a big bag of apples and crunch your way through as many as you want during the day. Then, gradually return to your normal way of eating, remembering to keep at least 50 per cent (better, 75 per cent) of your foods raw. Eating this way, we have been able to completely avoid the ravages of time-zone travel, with the result that we arrive looking and feeling great, instead of worn out.

Although we are very careful not to take too much in our suitcase, we also make sure, particularly on long flights, that we have as many little comforts as possible. While we don't try to take all of this with us at once, here are the things we often put into our carry-on bag.

- **Fresh fruit** Much better than plane food. Eating fresh fruit not only lessens the blow of jet-lag – 30,000 ft up and miles from anywhere, it also comes as a welcome and refreshing relief to the high-tech man-made world you are sitting in.
- **Relaxing music** The perfect antidote to travel stress. Take along a portable cassette player and your favourite relaxing sounds, say, Baroque concertos or some 'new age' tapes.
- **Ear-plugs** To shut out the constant hum of the engines, not to mention the baby crying, man snoring or lady chattering next to you. (The foam variety are better than the wax.)
- **Light fragrance** Refreshing when you need a lift.
- **Herbal tranquillizers** Valerian or passiflora tablets can be a great help in making you feel as if you are above the clouds – even if you *are* stuck in an aluminium plane.
- **Anti-stress formula** A high-potency B-complex vitamin supplement.
- **Jet-set aminos** L-tyrosine for a pick-up at your destination. L-tryptophan for when you need to sleep, but find it hard because of the time change.
- **Sleeping mask** An excellent complement to ear-plugs for blocking out the outside world and drifting into your own space.
- **Herbal tea sachets** Get the hostess to make it for you instead of the usual dreadful tea or coffee.
- **Good moisturizer** To counteract the dehydrating plane atmosphere and combat the stress on skin.
- **Ionizer** If you are lucky enough to have a portable one that's battery operated, it is a great way to overcome the negative effects of plane air.

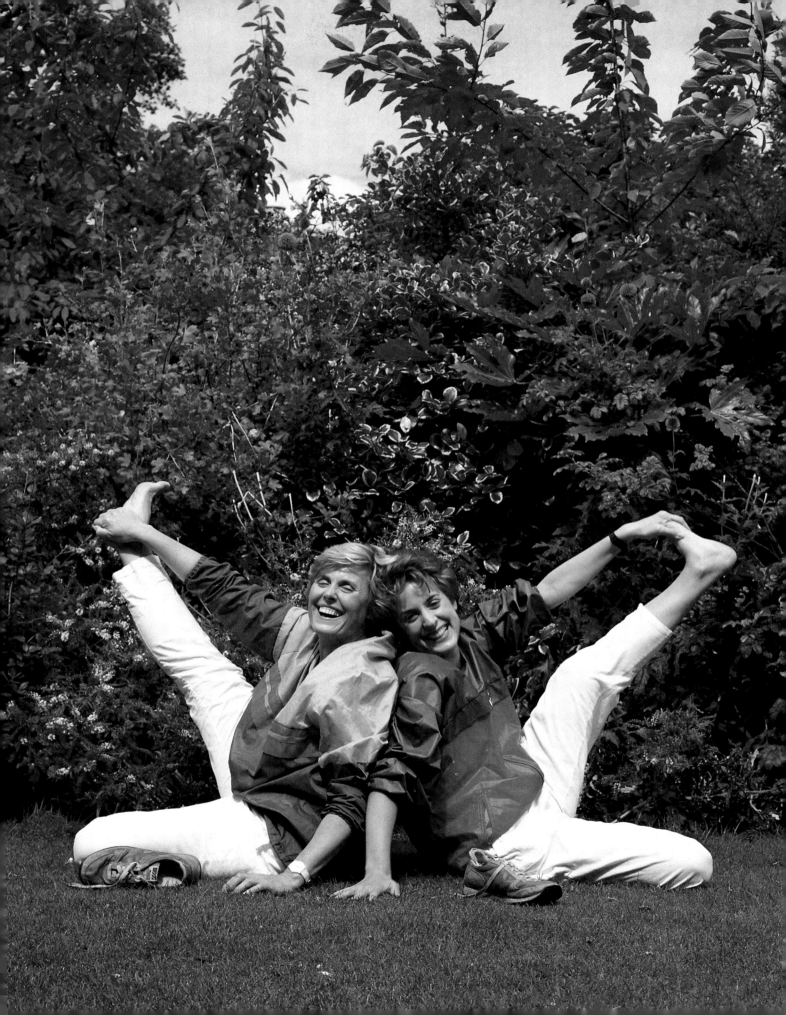

Index

ACKNOWLEDGEMENTS

The publishers wish to thank the following individuals and organizations for their help in the preparation of this book:

Butler and Wilson for jewellery; Chanel Boutique for jewellery; Paul Edmonds of 'Edmonds' for hair styling; Frances Hathaway for make-up; Alan Herdman for guidance during photography for the Pilates exercises; Nature's Best Health Products Ltd.

They also thank the following photographers and organizations for their kind permission to reproduce the photographs in this book:

Ardea 139 top centre; Avenue (Bart van Leeuwen) 79; Biofotos 139 top left and top right, 139 above, 139 below, 139 bottom left and bottom right; Camera Press 13, 117; Cent Idées (Barbro/Garçon) 101 (Burgi/Garçon) 84, 99, 118 (Chabaneix/Garçon) 28, 36 (Duffas/ Schoumacher) 71 (Tisné/Garçon) 57, 69 below, 93; Conran Octopus (Robyn Beeche) 2, 4–5, 12, 22–23, 32–35, 39, 44, 49, 53, 61, 68, 86–91, 105, 113, 115, 141 (Carrie Branovan) 8, 46, 131; Harpers and Queen/Carrie Branovan 58, 110, 133, 135; The Image Bank 11; Leslie Kenton 14; La Maison de Marie Claire (Chabaneix/ Bayle) 123; Marie Claire (E Kohli) 83 (Martin/Saulnier) 17 (Sacha) 103; Marie France (François Pomepui) 85; Octopus Books Ltd (John Freeman) 80 (Paul Williams) 27, 106; Harry Smith Photographic Horticultural Collection 139 bottom centre; Top Agence 31; Transworld Feature Syndicate (UK) Ltd 19, 25, 26, 40–41, 60, 62, 67, 69 above, 72, 73, 75, 77, 120, 127, 128–129; photograph courtesy of Vichy UK Ltd 97.

Acknowledgements